sex
365

sex
365

a position for every day

LONDON, NEW YORK, MELBOURNE, MUNICH, DELHI

Editor Elizabeth Watson
Senior Editor Peter Jones
Managing Editor Adèle Hayward
Art Director Peter Luff
Publisher Stephanie Jackson
Written by Nicole Bailey

Designer Vicky Read
Senior Designer Vanessa Hamilton
Production Editor Ben Marcus
Production Controller Mandy Inness

First American Edition, 2008

Published in the United States by
DK Publishing
375 Hudson Street
New York, New York 10014

10 11   10 9 8

SD356—January 2008

Published in Great Britain by Dorling Kindersley Limited

A catalog record for this book is available from the Library of Congress.

ISBN: 978-0-7566-3353-0

DK books are available at special discounts when purchased in bulk for sales promotions, premiums, fund-raising, or educational use. For details, contact: DK Publishing Special Markets, 375 Hudson Street, New York, New York 10014 or SpecialSales@dk.com.

PUBLISHER'S NOTE
Neither the publisher nor the author is engaged in rendering professional advice or services to the individual reader, and neither shall be liable or responsible for any loss or damage allegedly arising from any information or suggestion in this book. All participants in such activities must assume the responsibility for their own actions and safety and for compliance with all applicable laws. If you have any health problems or medical conditions or any other concerns about whether you are able to participate in any of these activities, you should take appropriate precautions. The information contained in this book cannot replace professional advice or sound judgment and good decision making, nor does the scope of this book allow for disclosure of all the potential hazards and risks involved in such activities.

Color reproduction by Colourscan in Singapore
Printed and bound in Singapore by Star Standard

Discover more at **www.dk.com**

introduction

Scratching your head for a sex position? Tired of the way he always goes on top? Need to wow a new lover? Driven to insane boredom by the spoons position? Want to try the sexual equivalent of a yoga workout? If you answer "yes" to one or more of these questions, *Sex 365* is for you. It exposes you to sex in all its naughty, saucy varieties. It's twisted sex, sex flipped upside-down, sex brought to its knees, and sex strung up from a bar. You can gape at the sex positions. You can marvel at them. You can even TRY them.

But before you embark on your year-long position-athon, remember the following things:

- Sex is great but don't forget to work, wash, and eat.
- Outdoor sex is hot, but do NOT get caught. Police stations aren't sexy. (Unless you like uniforms…).
- If it hurts, stop doing it. There's never any point in throwing your back (or anything else) out in the pursuit of novelty.
- Almost any position can be made easier with a super-sized tube of lube and some soft cushions.

Now just lie back and wrap your calves around your lover's head. Prepare to be rocked and rolled.

The positions

1   Spa treatment

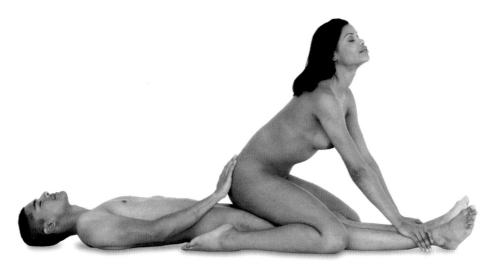

BEST FOR: sex in a private sauna
HITS THE SPOT FOR: salty, sweat-mingling passion
HOT TIP: let your hands skate across her back and butt

The director's chair   **2** ____

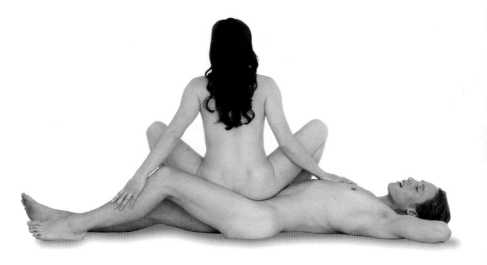

BEST FOR: when she wants to call the shots ————
HITS THE SPOT FOR: the thrill of her being in charge
HOT TIP: girls—lean back, put your hands on the floor, and jerk your hips

3   The cosmopolitan

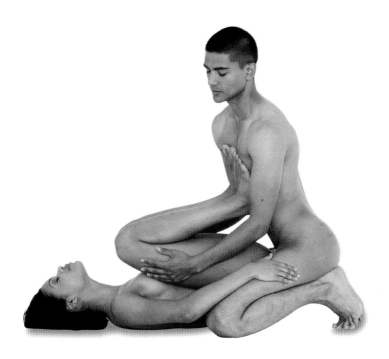

BEST FOR: hot one-night stands
HITS THE SPOT FOR: feeling the weight of his lust
HOT TIP: alternate fast, shallow strokes with slow, deep ones

Making hay while the sun shines

4 ___

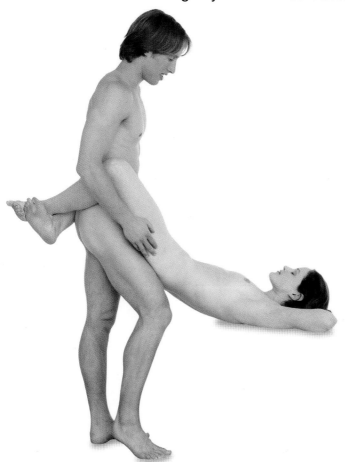

BEST FOR: sex off the end of a sun lounger ⎯⎯
HITS THE SPOT FOR: getting so worked up you splash sweat
HOT TIP: lovingly wash each other in the shower afterward

5 Under arrest

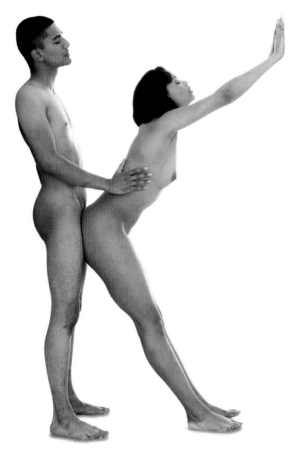

BEST FOR: sex with the sauciness of power play
HITS THE SPOT FOR: pretending that she's committed a criminal offense
HOT TIP: frisk her with her hands against the wall

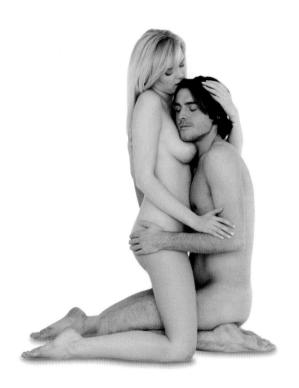

BEST FOR: dominatrixes in waiting
HITS THE SPOT FOR: giving him some very firm instruction
HOT TIP: order him to play with your nipples

7   Fancy meeting you here

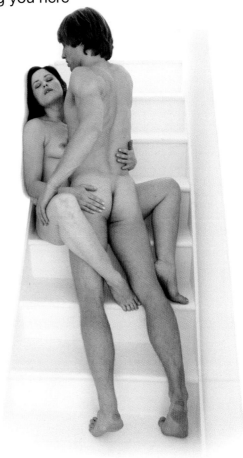

BEST FOR: impromptu encounters on the fire escape
HITS THE SPOT FOR: the kick of drop-your-pants, hitch-up-your-skirt sex
HOT TIP: girls—spread your knees wide and pull him into you

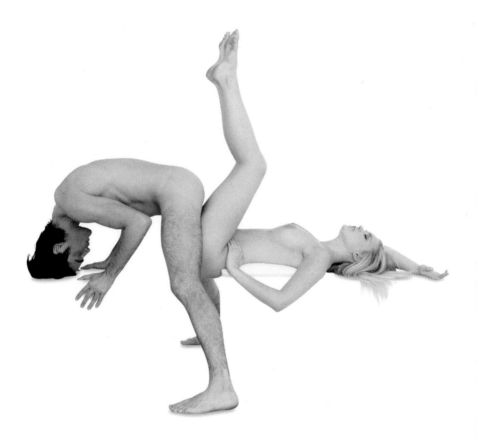

BEST FOR: when he wants to see a porn-style close-up
HITS THE SPOT FOR: getting an eyeful of the action
HOT TIP: it looks even hotter if she masturbates

9   The half frog

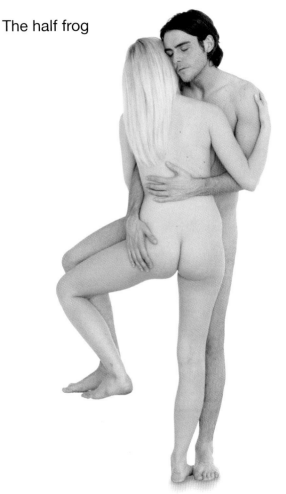

BEST FOR: when you want to cuddle, stroke, caress, and press
HITS THE SPOT FOR: getting inside each other's skin
HOT TIP: substitute the block for the edge of a bed

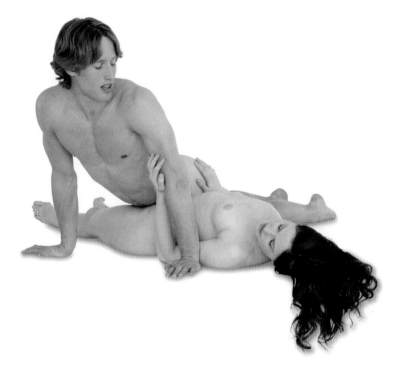

BEST FOR: "we're-between-positions" sex
HITS THE SPOT FOR: novel penis-bending sensations
HOT TIP: move from this position into The look-out (see 104)

11 The dreamer

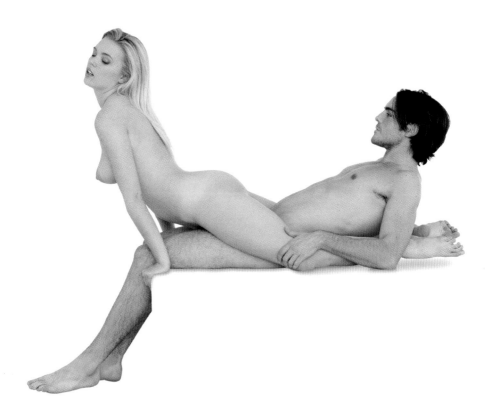

BEST FOR: men who love bottoms
HITS THE SPOT FOR: her taking control
HOT TIP: men — lie back and take in the view

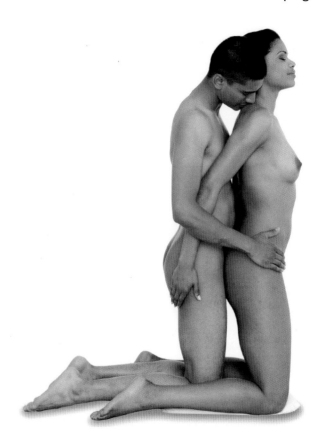

BEST FOR: when he shuffles up unannounced
HITS THE SPOT FOR: bringing you to your knees (if you weren't there already)
HOT TIP: keep your hands busy at all times

13 Standing room only

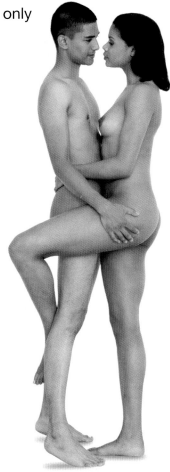

BEST FOR: sex in the supply closet
HITS THE SPOT FOR: the erotic thrill that someone might open the door
HOT TIP: girls—wear a short skirt for fast access

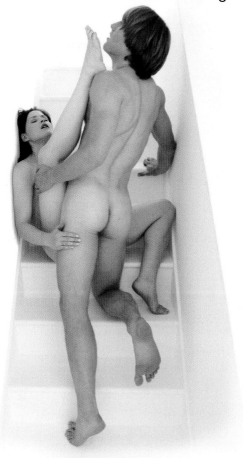

BEST FOR: when you probably shouldn't be doing it
HITS THE SPOT FOR: feeling naughty yet excited
HOT TIP: set a time to do it all over again

15 Oasis

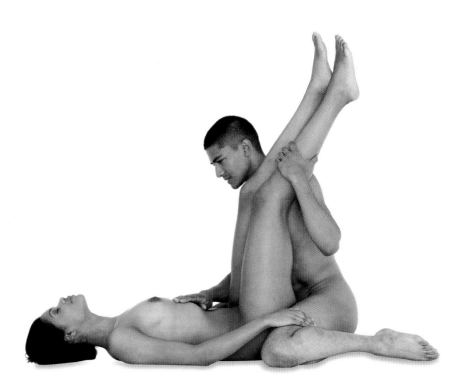

BEST FOR: leg men
HITS THE SPOT FOR: being close, and yet so far
HOT TIP: her legs should be as smooth as a baby's bottom

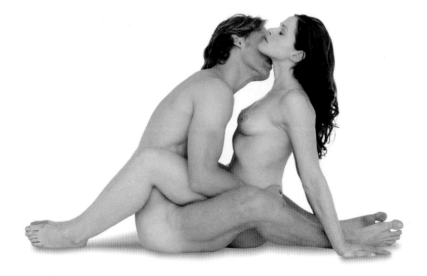

BEST FOR: we-can't-bear-to-be-apart sex
HITS THE SPOT FOR: the ecstasy of long passionate kisses
HOT TIP: imagine you're the only two people in the world

17 Standing 69

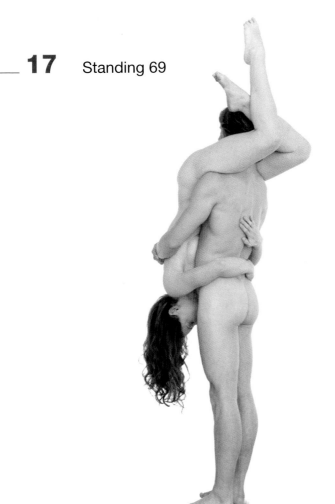

BEST FOR: an experience you won't forget
HITS THE SPOT FOR: the thrill of being able to say you've done it
HOT TIP: pick her up when she's on the bed with her head off the edge

Domestic harlot **18** _____

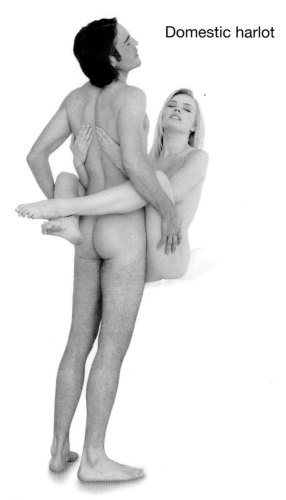

BEST FOR: sex on the washing machine ——
HITS THE SPOT FOR: making you smile while you're at it
HOT TIP: set the washing machine to the spin cycle

19   The sharp shooter

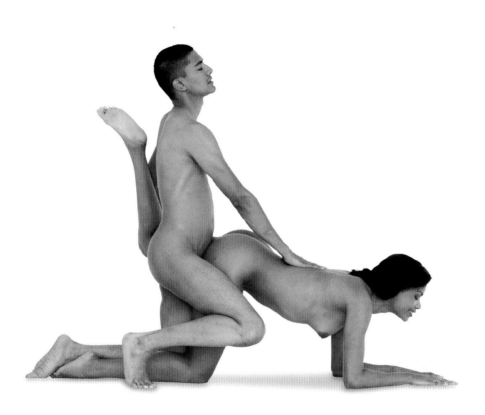

BEST FOR: when you're aiming for a position-a-thon
HITS THE SPOT FOR: a few in and out strokes before moving swiftly on
HOT TIP: start and finish with her on all fours

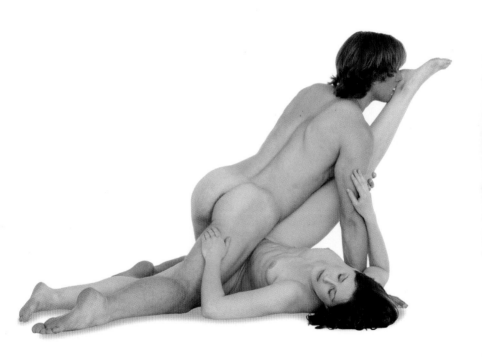

BEST FOR: guys with a foot fetish

HITS THE SPOT FOR: planting make-you-melt kisses on her ankles

HOT TIP: take the opportunity to fondle his thigh and buttock

21 Dirty dancing

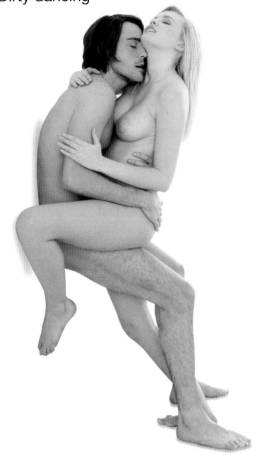

BEST FOR: when dancing gets so hot it turns into sex
HITS THE SPOT FOR: sating lust that can't be ignored for another second
HOT TIP: whisper breathlessly "I want you"

Three-tool massage **22**

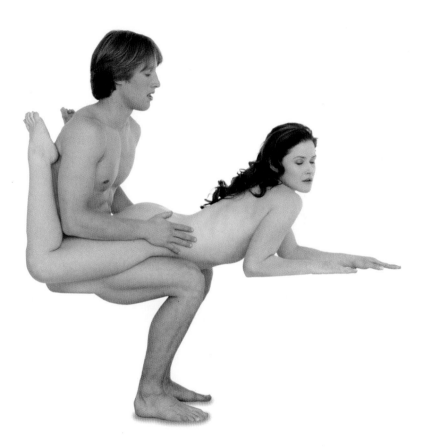

BEST FOR: backrub plus penetration
HITS THE SPOT FOR: triple-loaded pampering for her
HOT TIP: include her B-side in the massage too

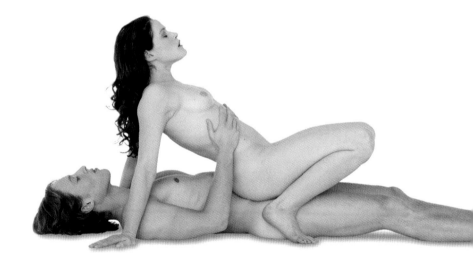

BEST FOR: sex that's elegant, erotic, and sensual
HITS THE SPOT FOR: tickling his chest with her hair
HOT TIP: burn incense and let the smoke waft over you

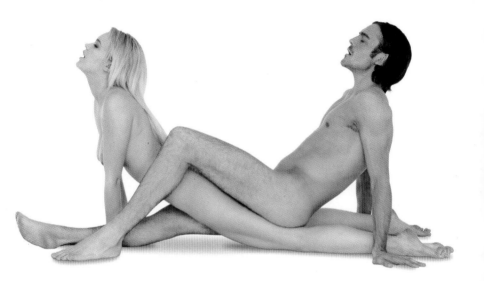

BEST FOR: funny, playful foreplay ___
HITS THE SPOT FOR: sliding his buttocks over hers
HOT TIP: try the same with her on top

25 The invitation

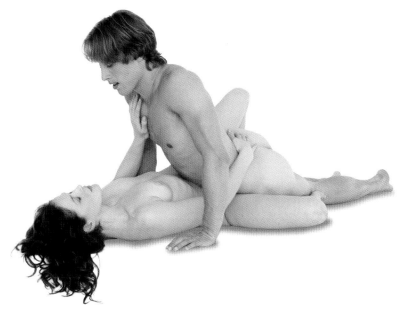

BEST FOR: lazy and languorous "we've-got-all-day" sex
HITS THE SPOT FOR: gazing into each others' eyes
HOT TIP: try it on a rug in front of a log fire

The inverted wheelbarrow **26**

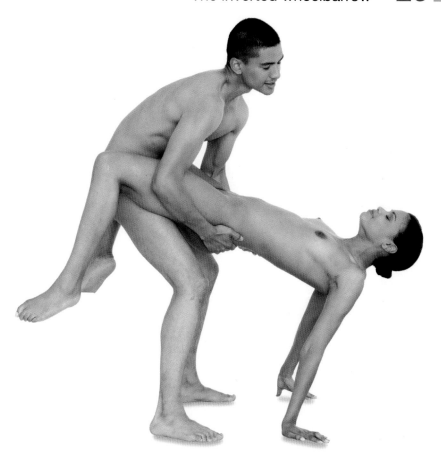

BEST FOR: lovers who enjoy sexercise
HITS THE SPOT FOR: her feeling widely opened
HOT TIP: be a gentleman—take most of her weight in your arms

27   Kneel, straddle, hook, and clasp

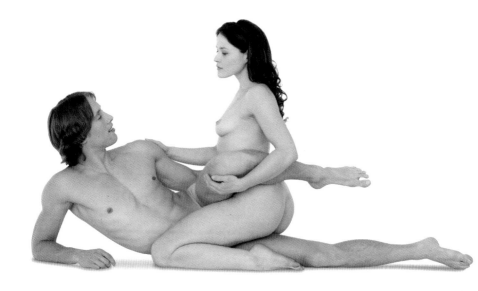

BEST FOR: a non-penetrative option (i.e., when you forgot the condoms)
HITS THE SPOT FOR: her humping his thigh
HOT TIP: a 69 is another safe option

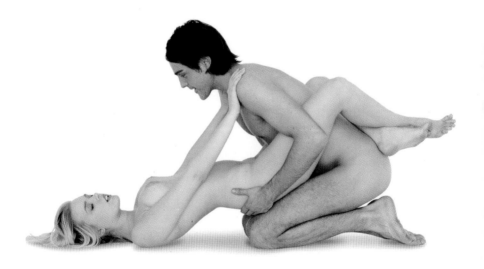

BEST FOR: passionate, hungry sex
HITS THE SPOT FOR: speedy relief when you haven't done it in a while
HOT TIP: get super-aroused by picturing it in your head beforehand

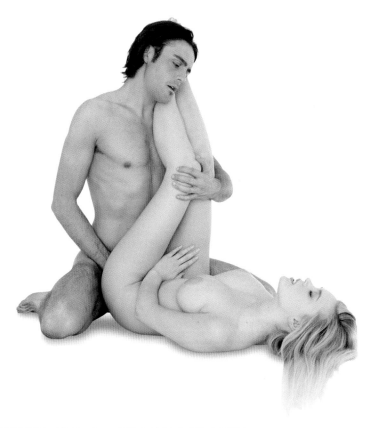

BEST FOR: when you want a slow guided entry
HITS THE SPOT FOR: making her tremble with anticipation
HOT TIP: guys—pull out mid-sex, and swirl your penis tip around her clitoris

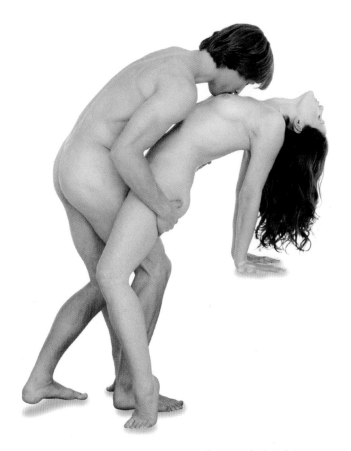

BEST FOR: he-sends-her-into-a-swoon sex
HITS THE SPOT FOR: expressing strong and silent virility
HOT TIP: picture yourselves in *Gone with the Wind*

31   Palm to palm

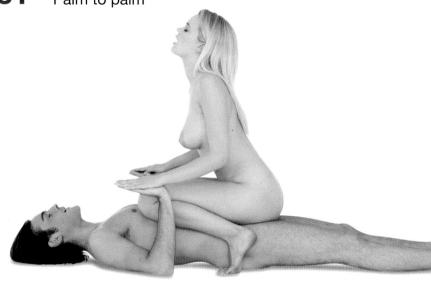

BEST FOR: when the neighbors are out and can't hear you
HITS THE SPOT FOR: friction in all the right places for both of you
HOT TIP: shout when you're tipping over the edge

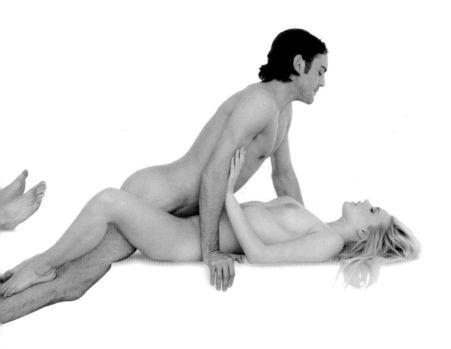

BEST FOR: a quickie before work
HITS THE SPOT FOR: distracting you while you're getting up
HOT TIP: try it off the edge of the bed with your underwear on

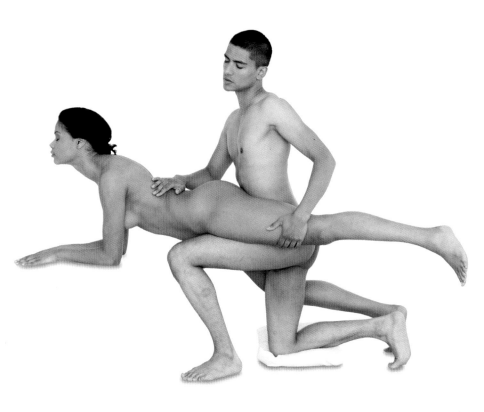

BEST FOR: a quickie during the commercial break
HITS THE SPOT FOR: delicate fingertip caresses on her back and buttocks
HOT TIP: guys—unless you've got a cast-iron knee, put a pillow on the floor

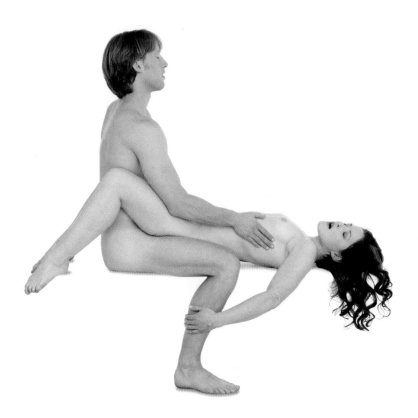

BEST FOR: women who get crazy on breast play
HITS THE SPOT FOR: making her wild and breathless
HOT TIP: tweak, stroke, flick, fondle, brush, and cup. Don't forget the baby oil

35 Stand and deliver

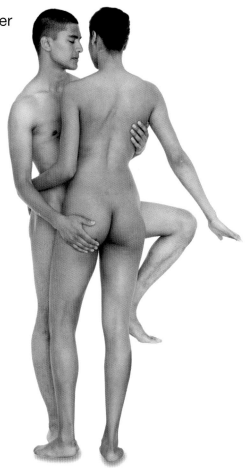

BEST FOR: when your dinner guests are in the other room
HITS THE SPOT FOR: giving her sexy little buttock squeezes
HOT TIP: guys — squat a little if you want to enter her

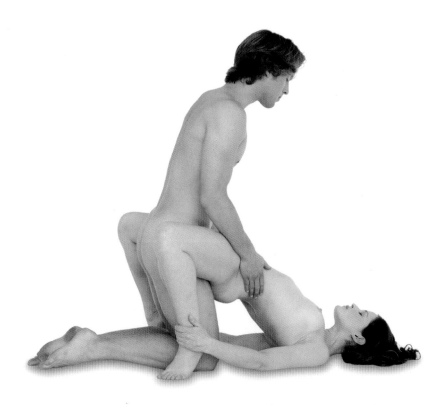

BEST FOR: women with flexible backs ———
HITS THE SPOT FOR: giggling after a head rush
HOT TIP: remember the firm helping hand around her waist

37 Undertow

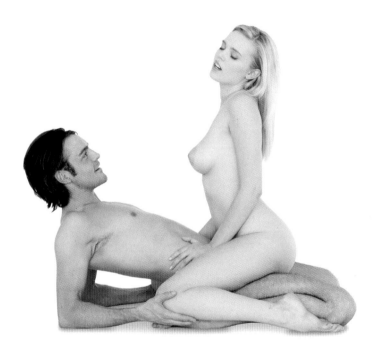

BEST FOR: when she needs a good and proper servicing
HITS THE SPOT FOR: giving her a raised platform to ride and glide on
HOT TIP: ladies—flick those hips

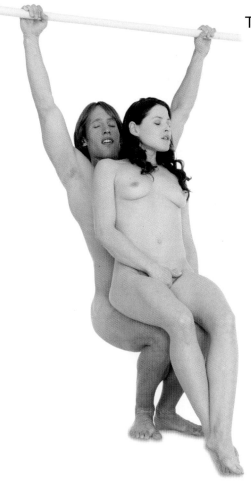

BEST FOR: gentlemanly sex that puts her first
HITS THE SPOT FOR: her touching herself the way she wants
HOT TIP: get strong muscles so you can stay in position until she comes

39 Just add leather

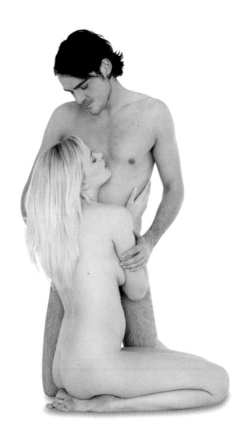

BEST FOR: BDSM dabblers in kinky leather harnesses
HITS THE SPOT FOR: making him feel all-powerful and her feel all helpless
HOT TIP: handcuff her wrists, then describe the fantasy you'd like to act out

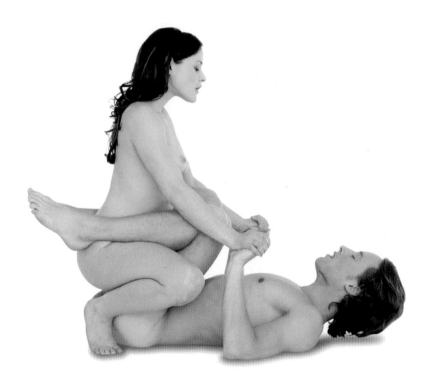

BEST FOR: when she's bursting with energy
HITS THE SPOT FOR: working off a backlog of sexual tension
HOT TIP: girls—explore your masculine side. Take control

41 Interior decorator

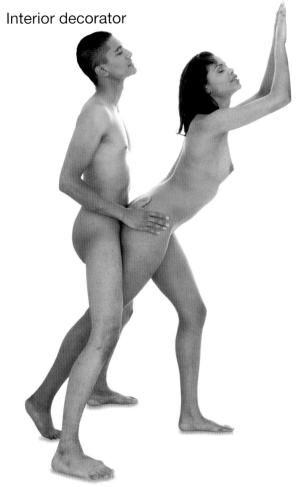

BEST FOR: when you want a smooth coverage and a high-quality finish
HITS THE SPOT FOR: perfecting your brush strokes
HOT TIP: watch the wet, glossy movements of your penis

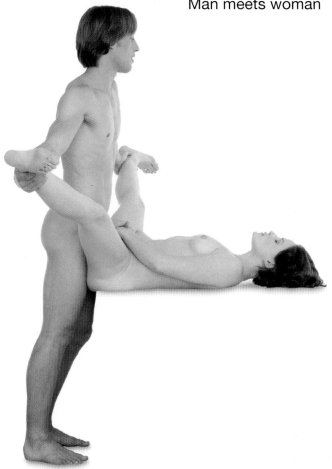

BEST FOR: hard and fast, genital-jolting passion
HITS THE SPOT FOR: rhythmic fingers-on-clitoris action for her
HOT TIP: get your bits at exactly the same altitude

43 Thigh hook

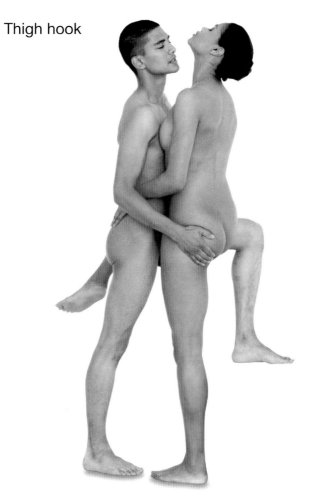

BEST FOR: a quickie in the bathroom—he rests his foot on the bathtub
HITS THE SPOT FOR: that intimate "locked together" feeling
HOT TIP: guide him in and out using leg pressure

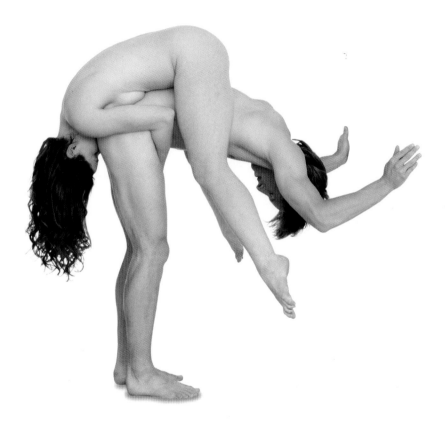

BEST FOR: the super-sexpert approach to rimming your lover

HITS THE SPOT FOR: feeling like a sexual pioneer

HOT TIP: have some cushions nearby in case she falls off

45 Lady of leisure

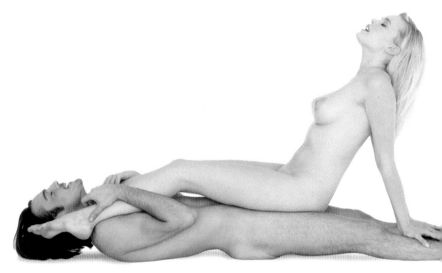

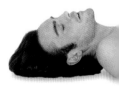

BEST FOR: women who love being on top
HITS THE SPOT FOR: taking your time to work up to a delicious climax
HOT TIP: grip his shoulders with your feet and move yourself back and forth

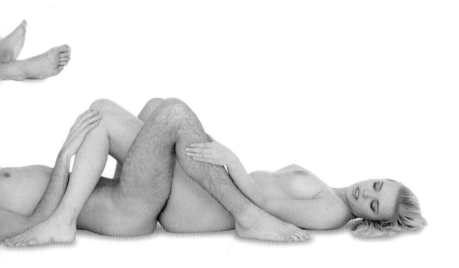

BEST FOR: when you lie back after climaxing

HITS THE SPOT FOR: savoring the after-tremors of orgasm while still joined

HOT TIP: raise and lower your hips in sync

47 The manhandle-her

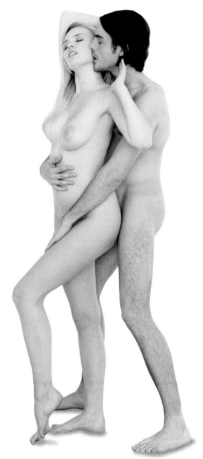

BEST FOR: while you're waiting for the wine to cool
HITS THE SPOT FOR: pressing all of her buttons at once
HOT TIP: give him feedback such as "harder" or "faster." Or just "mmmm…"

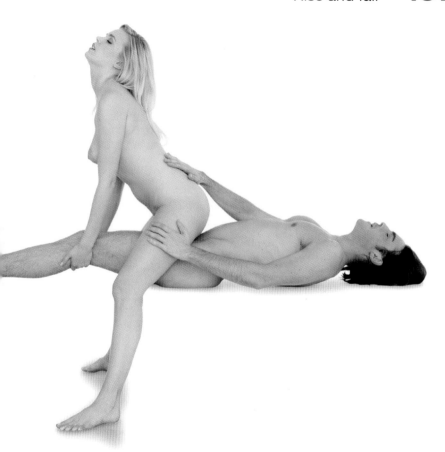

BEST FOR: girls who want to get their thighs trim ————
HITS THE SPOT FOR: achieving a warm, wet, satisfying rhythm
HOT TIP: stand, squat, stand, squat, and…dooooon't stop

49 Gym queen

BEST FOR: after-hours sex at your local gym
HITS THE SPOT FOR: enjoying stand-up sex without the weight
HOT TIP: girls—let your head drop back and enjoy the ride

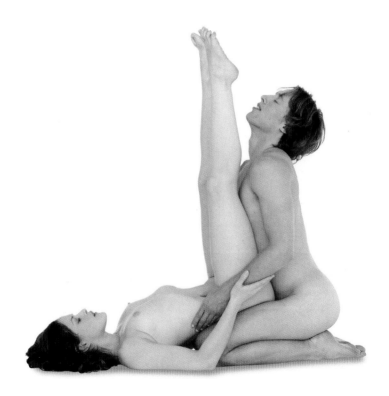

BEST FOR: a glorious follow-up to cunnilingus

HITS THE SPOT FOR: his glans gently pressing toward her cervix

HOT TIP: guys—devote yourself to her pleasure

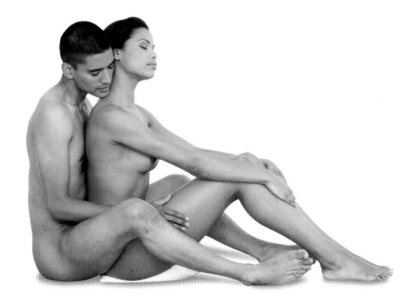

BEST FOR: sex in the tub

HITS THE SPOT FOR: no one getting landed with the faucet end

HOT TIP: girls—wiggle your bottom backward until you can feel his erection

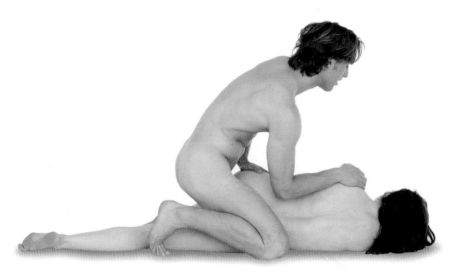

BEST FOR: when he can't decide which entrance to go through
HITS THE SPOT FOR: a little light anal penetration
HOT TIP: anal sex is easier if she bears down as he enters

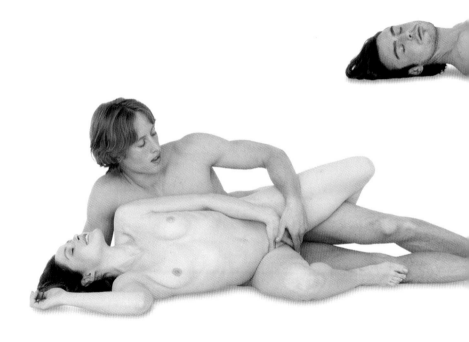

BEST FOR: when she wants to put her finger on the button
HITS THE SPOT FOR: getting her off quickly
HOT TIP: two hands are better than one

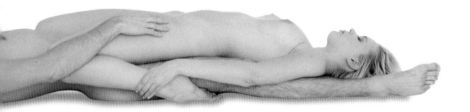

BEST FOR: chilled-out sex for laid-back lovers
HITS THE SPOT FOR: gazing dreamily at the clouds
HOT TIP: lazily caress the bits of each other you can get your hands on

55 The push-off

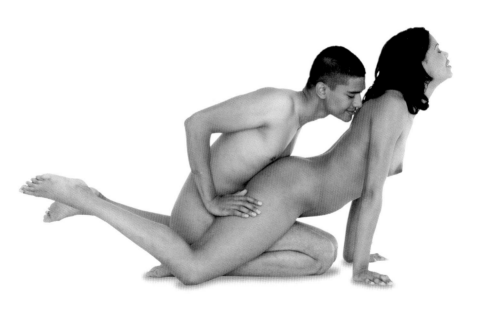

BEST FOR: when you're fueled ready for take-off
HITS THE SPOT FOR: G-spot pressure to die for
HOT TIP: blow on the back of her neck or her spine

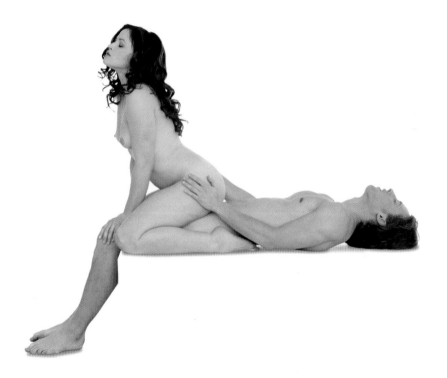

BEST FOR: blindfolded sex

HITS THE SPOT FOR: freeing you both from inhibition

HOT TIP: make up for the lack of visuals with some passionate moaning

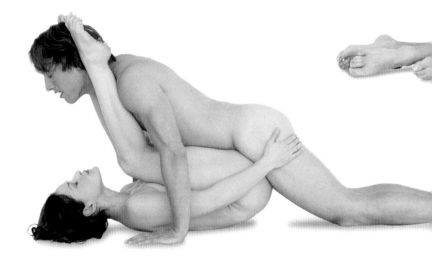

BEST FOR: flexible women (in more ways than one)
HITS THE SPOT FOR: being big on intensity and big on intimacy
HOT TIP: make this your climax scene rather than your first act

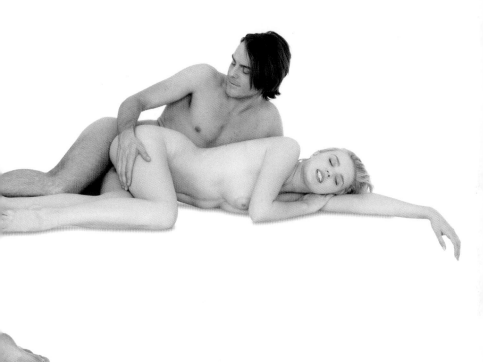

BEST FOR: inconspicuous sex under a blanket

HITS THE SPOT FOR: naughty, clandestine thrills

HOT TIP: if you hear someone coming—no, not you—fain sleep

59 The accommodator

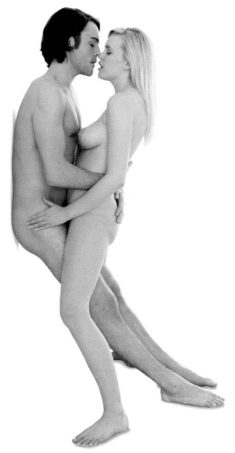

BEST FOR: standing-up sex when she's shorter than him
HITS THE SPOT FOR: comfort in a compact space
HOT TIP: work in harmony to get a rhythm going

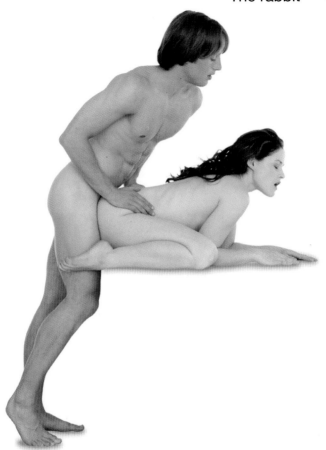

BEST FOR: easy-entry anal sex

HITS THE SPOT FOR: deep, intense, shuddering orgasms

HOT TIP: practice with a finger if you're an anal novice

61 Butter on hot toast

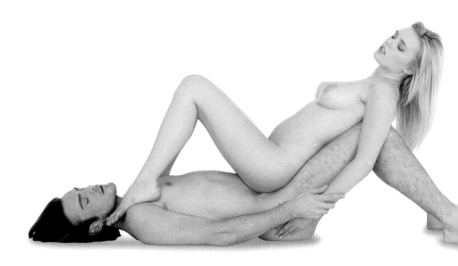

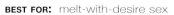

BEST FOR: melt-with-desire sex
HITS THE SPOT FOR: plenty of skin-on-skin sliding sensations
HOT TIP: ladies—lean back and let his legs support your weight

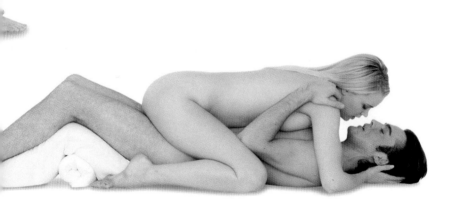

BEST FOR: when his back's not working but his love muscle is

HITS THE SPOT FOR: achieving that convalescent climax

HOT TIP: ladies—think light; think gentle

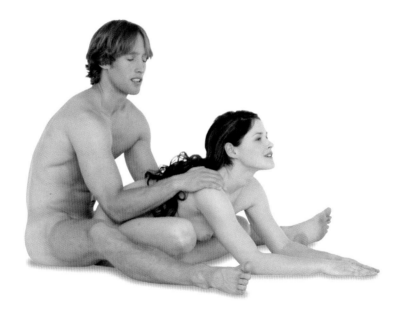

BEST FOR: the end of a long, stressful day
HITS THE SPOT FOR: a shoulder massage that makes her dissolve
HOT TIP: guys—when the time is right, lift her onto your waiting erection

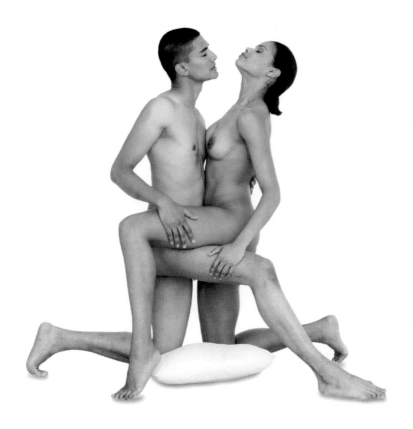

BEST FOR: when you're feeling strong and sturdy
HITS THE SPOT FOR: burning arousal as you thump into each other
HOT TIP: stand with your penis between her breasts, then sink to your knee

65 Desert lion

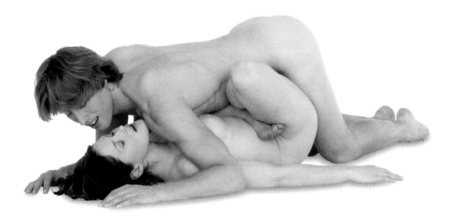

BEST FOR: women who can do the lotus position—and hold it
HITS THE SPOT FOR: erotic bondage sensations
HOT TIP: use straps and handcuffs for an easier bondage fix

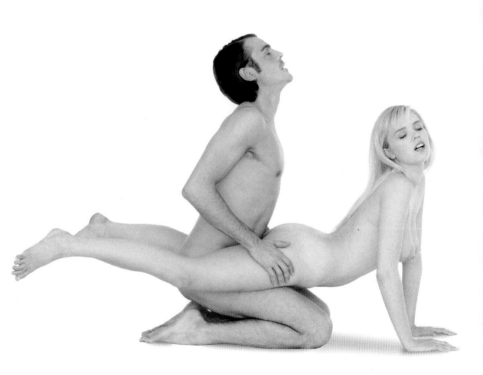

BEST FOR: sex in shallow water
HITS THE SPOT FOR: lapping sensations on her G-spot
HOT TIP: try it on a deserted beach as the tide comes in

67 Corridor coitus

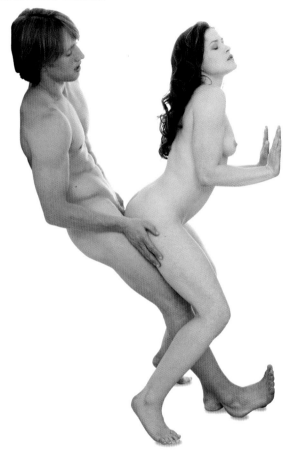

BEST FOR: when you've just invited her in for "coffee"
HITS THE SPOT FOR: the hot thrill of impulsive sex
HOT TIP: don't say "would you like cream with that?"

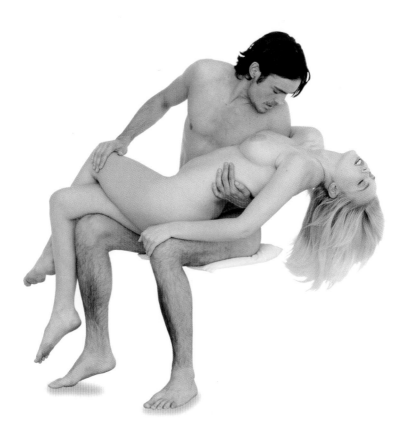

BEST FOR: weak-with-lust, carry-me-to-bed-now sex
HITS THE SPOT FOR: making up your own porn-style plot
HOT TIP: create a sex den in which to enact your drama

69 Just add one

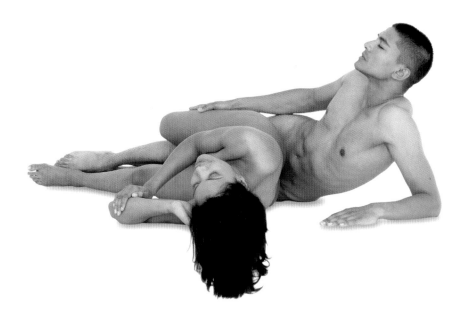

BEST FOR: threesomes
HITS THE SPOT FOR: earning your stars as brazen sexperimenters
HOT TIP: the third party lies on his/her side facing her—the rest is up to you

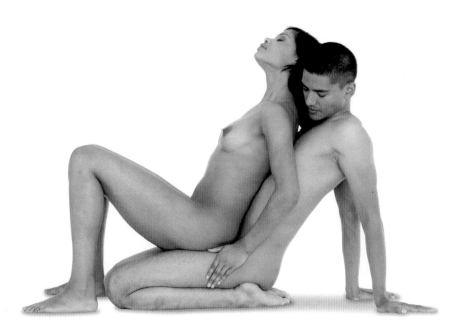

BEST FOR: women in search of their G-spot
HITS THE SPOT FOR: her thinking: "wow, I never felt that before"
HOT TIP: massage her G-spot with your fingers first—yes, it's the first ridge

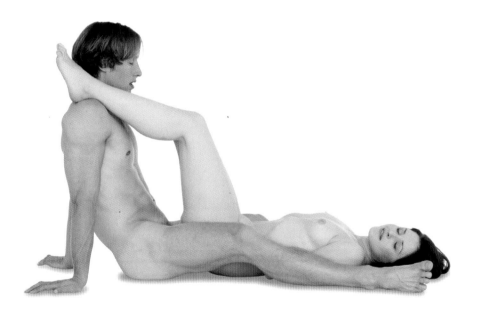

BEST FOR: in a field of tall waving grass
HITS THE SPOT FOR: being inconspicuous
HOT TIP: dress with the possibility of grass stains in mind

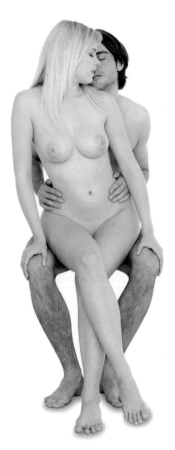

BEST FOR: pretending she's just sitting on his lap

HITS THE SPOT FOR: the hot thrill of sex in public

HOT TIP: wear easy-access clothes…oh, and don't get caught

73   Is this seat taken?

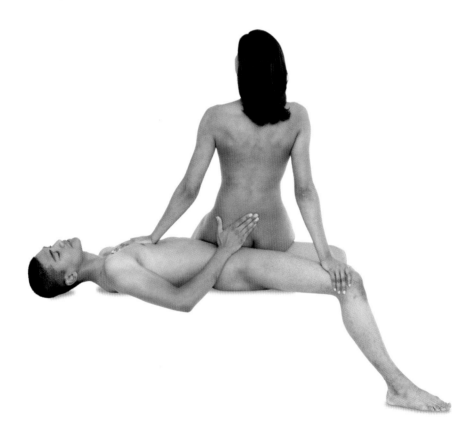

BEST FOR: kinky role play
HITS THE SPOT FOR: pretending you don't know each other
HOT TIP: keep the role play going afterward

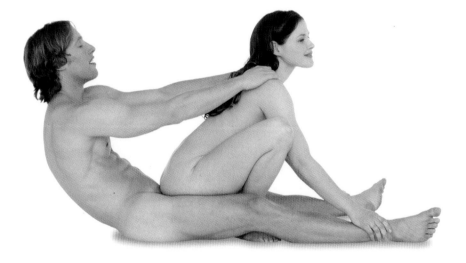

BEST FOR: sex in a rowboat
HITS THE SPOT FOR: feeling like you're really working as a team
HOT TIP: if you haven't got a rowboat, do it in the bathtub

75 The raised rabbit

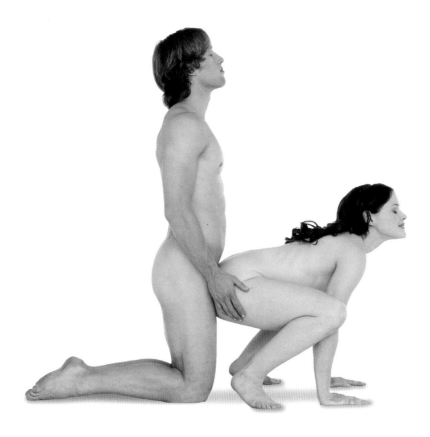

BEST FOR: the raunchy "we know what we're doing" variety of anal sex
HITS THE SPOT FOR: going in deep
HOT TIP: if you're well endowed, enter in slowly

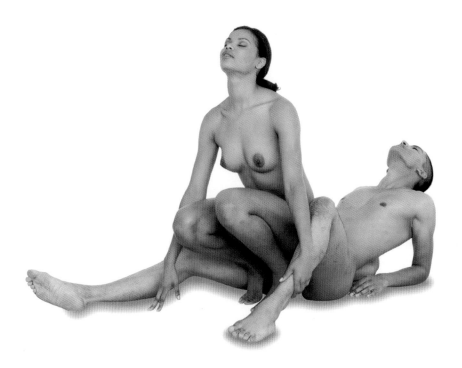

BEST FOR: "Good evening. Can I help you with that erection sir?" sex

HITS THE SPOT FOR: the thrill of flirty "stranger" sex

HOT TIP: book into a real hotel and dress the part

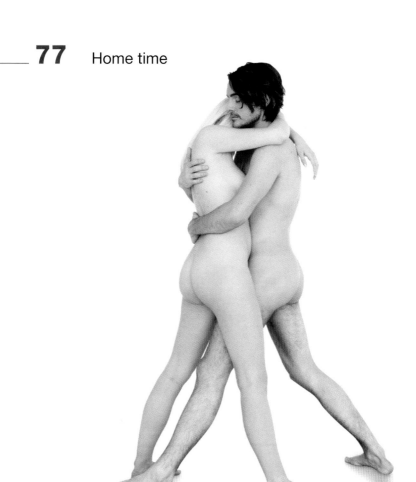

BEST FOR: foreplay at the end of a drunken party
HITS THE SPOT FOR: enjoying a smooch while also propping each other up
HOT TIP: call for a taxi first

Behind you all the way 78

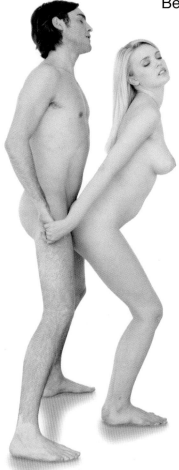

BEST FOR: sex on hotel balconies
HITS THE SPOT FOR: the oh-so-naughty delight of a public quickie
HOT TIP: keep most of your clothes on—and keep a straight face

79   X marks the spot

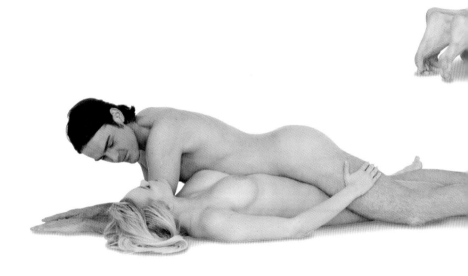

BEST FOR: discovering her hidden treasure
HITS THE SPOT FOR: intense clitoris friction as her legs are close together
HOT TIP: keep your shaft moving fast and parallel to her clitoris

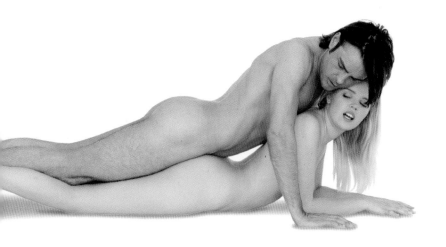

BEST FOR: spontaneous sofa-sex
HITS THE SPOT FOR: the tip of his glans gliding against her G-spot
HOT TIP: girls—push your ass up toward him

81 Creep up behind me

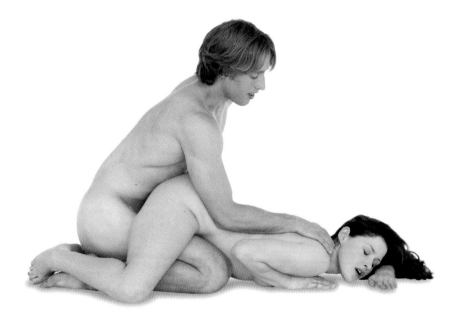

BEST FOR: lovers exploring the darker side of sex
HITS THE SPOT FOR: fulfilling her "do what you want with me" fantasies
HOT TIP: go the whole nine yards and dress in bondage gear

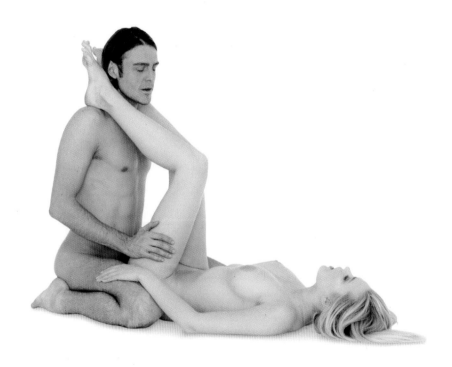

BEST FOR: men who are "cliterate"
HITS THE SPOT FOR: his thumb swirling and circling on her clitoris
HOT TIP: kiss the soles of her feet

83 The barmaid

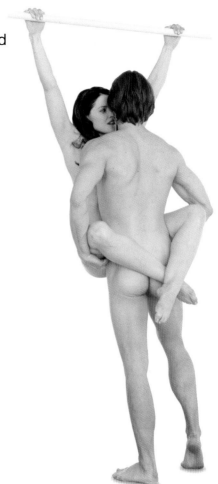

BEST FOR: when she wants to give him a sound servicing
HITS THE SPOT FOR: hot skin-to-skin contact
HOT TIP: guys—grab her squarely and move her on and off you

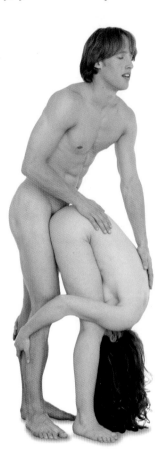

BEST FOR: when she feels faint
HITS THE SPOT FOR: giving him a powerful erection
HOT TIP: when her knees are this close to her ears, penetration is deep

85 Love knot

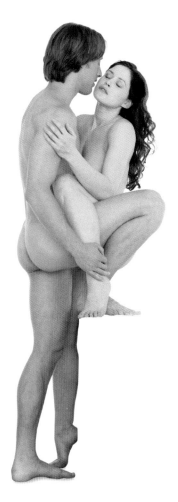

BEST FOR: when you've got something romantic to whisper
HITS THE SPOT FOR: the joy of deep penetration while standing up
HOT TIP: you might not be able to move much, but relish the sensation

The half-shoulderstand   **86**

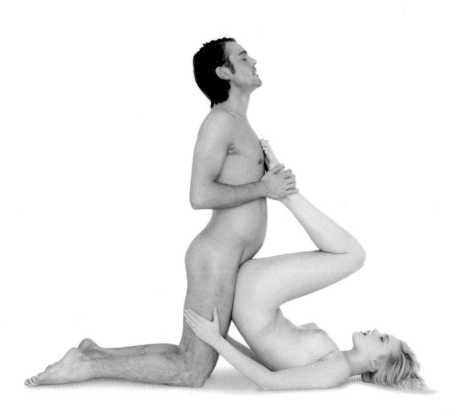

BEST FOR: gymnast aficionados
HITS THE SPOT FOR: guaranteeing a tight connection
HOT TIP: girls — show off by putting your knees on your forehead

87 Let me give you a leg up

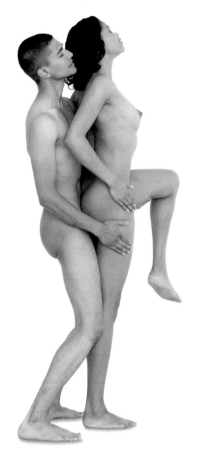

BEST FOR: lovers who don't mind falling over
HITS THE SPOT FOR: silly, sexy, spontaneous thrills
HOT TIP: topple over onto a bed or a sofa and keep going

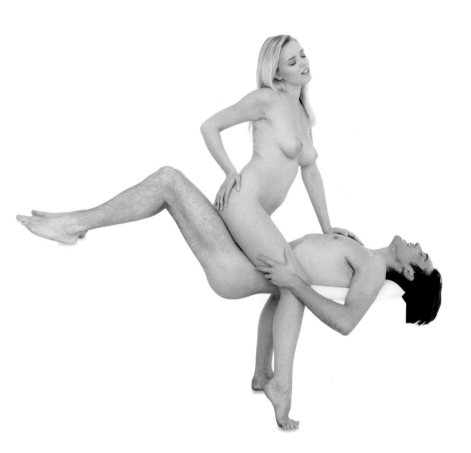

BEST FOR: men who find Come sit at my table (see 189) too strenuous
HITS THE SPOT FOR: the slick feel of her ass sliding up and down his thighs
HOT TIP: a bed and a nearby desk will work just as well

89 The deep dog

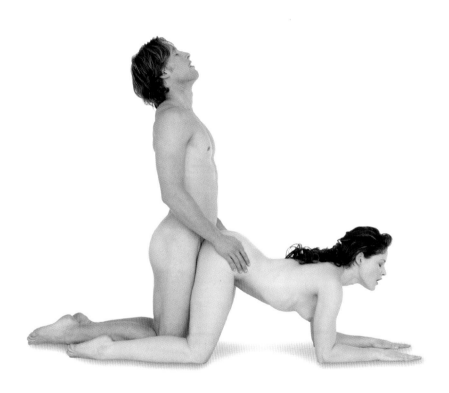

BEST FOR: ready and raw animalistic sex
HITS THE SPOT FOR: giving yourself up to sweaty, noisy passion
HOT TIP: thrust like there's no tomorrow

The restrained dog **90**

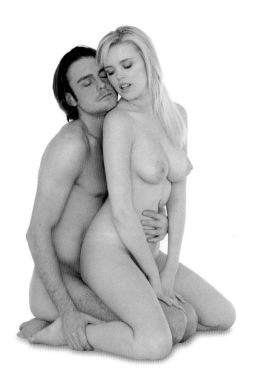

BEST FOR: when you've just been pounding away in The deep dog (left)

HITS THE SPOT FOR: gathering your energy before you go for the finish

HOT TIP: get two pairs of hands working on her front

91 The carpet burn

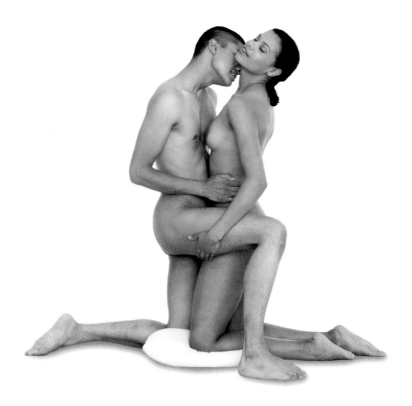

BEST FOR: getting give-away raw knees
HITS THE SPOT FOR: a reminder of what you did last night: raw knees = raw sex
HOT TIP: don't say to friends: "oh, I tripped going upstairs"

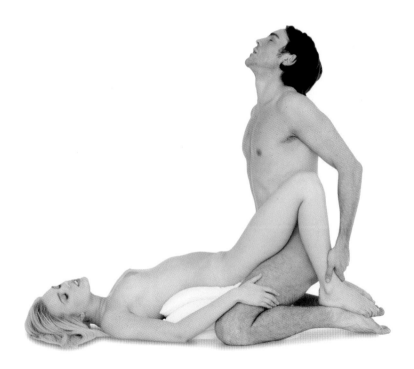

BEST FOR: when you want precision entry
HITS THE SPOT FOR: getting your genitals in perfect alignment
HOT TIP: put pillows, cushions, or a pile of towels underneath her

93 Z bed

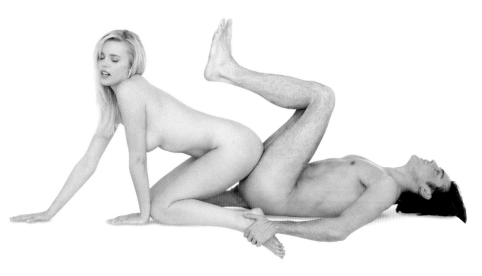

BEST FOR: some pre-sex teasing
HITS THE SPOT FOR: titillating but barely penetrating
HOT TIP: use your hand to guide your penis to her hot spots

The hanging gardens of Babylon **94**

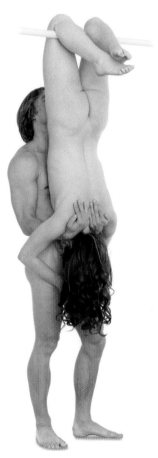

BEST FOR: the lightweight version of a standing 69
HITS THE SPOT FOR: getting the adrenaline pumping
HOT TIP: trapeze training helps

95 The insatiable

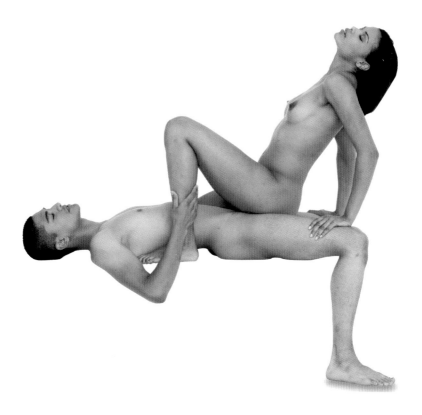

BEST FOR: seconds, thirds, or fourths
HITS THE SPOT FOR: getting into a powerful genital-mashing rhythm
HOT TIP: reach behind you to brush your fingertips lightly against his balls

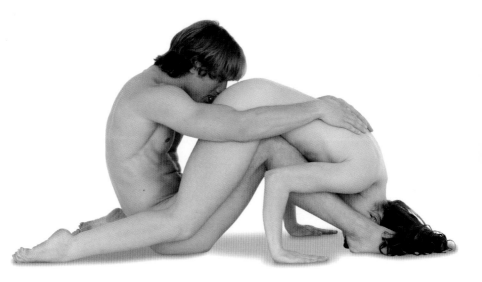

BEST FOR: oral sex in compact spaces
HITS THE SPOT FOR: swirling tongue action on her local beauty spots
HOT TIP: don't do it in the bathtub

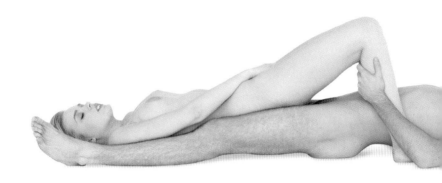

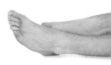

BEST FOR: when you've both just had a head-blasting orgasm
HITS THE SPOT FOR: lying back in post-coital bliss
HOT TIP: close your eyes and bask

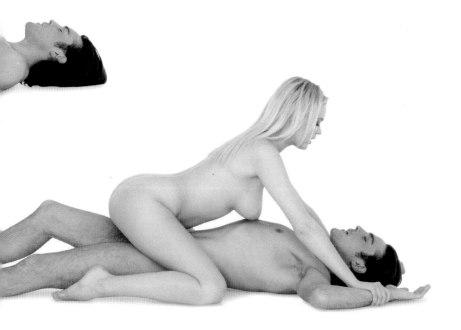

BEST FOR: full-on rutting when you're both H-O-T
HITS THE SPOT FOR: complete post-sex satiation
HOT TIP: pin his wrists to the ground for a frisson of S&M

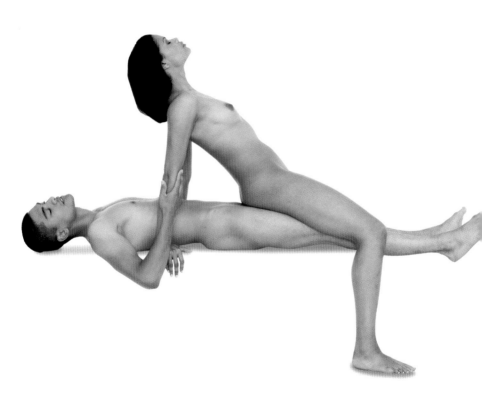

BEST FOR: hot sweaty nights when you don't want to be too close
HITS THE SPOT FOR: the intensity of her vagina hugging the length of his penis
HOT TIP: do mini pelvic thrusts on him

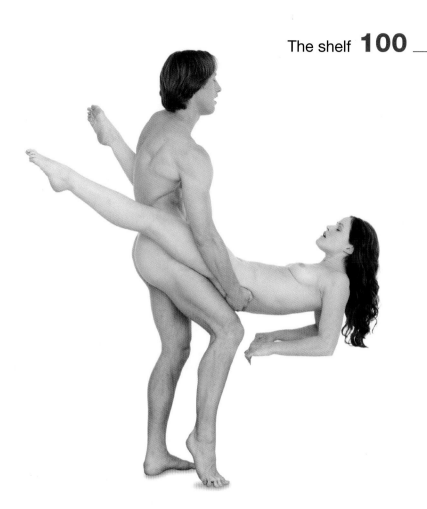

BEST FOR: lovers who want an advanced-sex challenge
HITS THE SPOT FOR: her showing off a super-toned body
HOT TIP: think of your elbows—wear pads

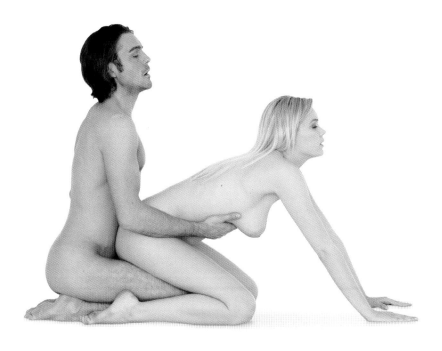

BEST FOR: those who want a gentler take on doggy style sex
HITS THE SPOT FOR: making you both whimper with pleasure
HOT TIP: wiggle your hips like you'd wag a tail

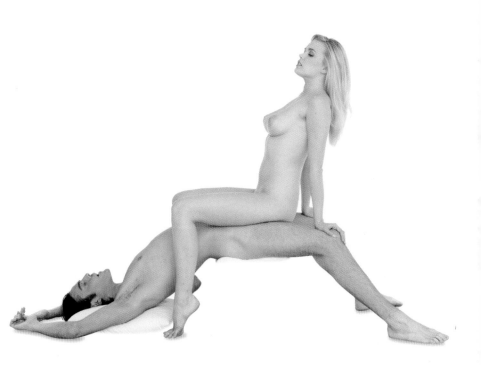

BEST FOR: use-him-and-abuse-him sex
HITS THE SPOT FOR: the special intoxication of submission
HOT TIP: girls—play up the role of dom

103 Vacation romance

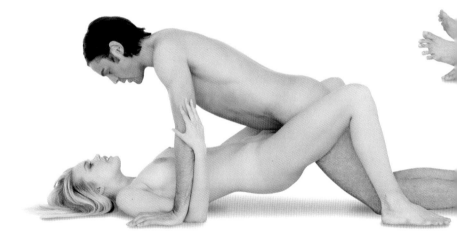

BEST FOR: balmy summer evenings
HITS THE SPOT FOR: mutual thrusting — he dips and she rises
HOT TIP: sip a margarita by the pool afterward

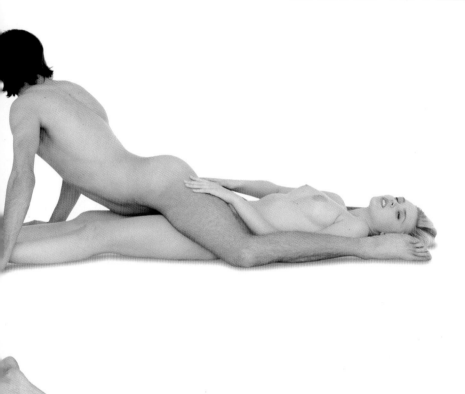

BEST FOR: anonymous-sex fantasies
HITS THE SPOT FOR: grazing your fingernails across his buttocks
HOT TIP: ever tried anal beads? Surprise him!

105 The bridge of sighs

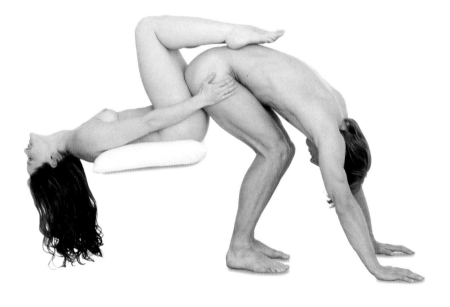

BEST FOR: elephantine penis owners
HITS THE SPOT FOR: giving her a small taste of the beast
HOT TIP: if you're over-endowed, this position will "minimize" you

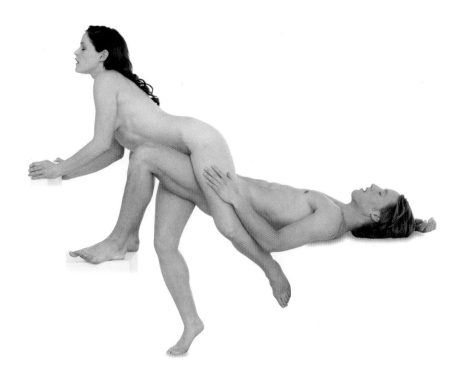

BEST FOR: when she's in the mood to tease rather than please ____
HITS THE SPOT FOR: moving up and down his thigh so your bits barely touch
HOT TIP: wait until he's sizzling before firmly impaling yourself on his shaft

107 Nostalgia for the 70s

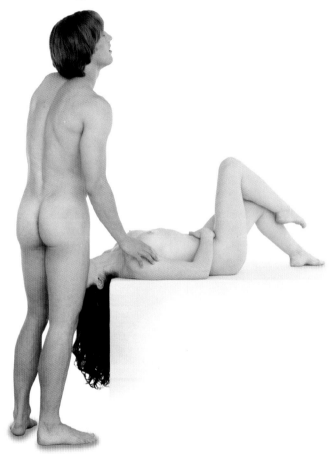

BEST FOR: lovers who want to try deep throat
HITS THE SPOT FOR: swallowing his sword up to the hilt
HOT TIP: relax your throat, guide him slowly, and remember to breathe!

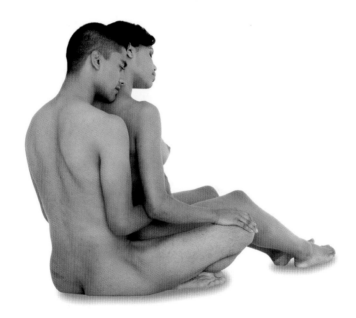

BEST FOR: lovers who like to meditate
HITS THE SPOT FOR: feeling at one with each other
HOT TIP: take long, slow, deep breaths together

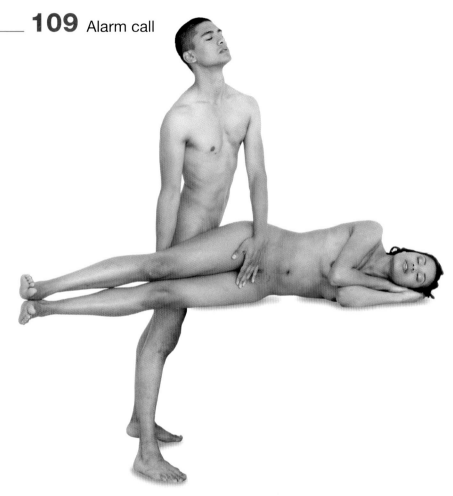

109 Alarm call

BEST FOR: when she's finding it hard to get up in the morning
HITS THE SPOT FOR: gently igniting desire
HOT TIP: stroke her body with yours

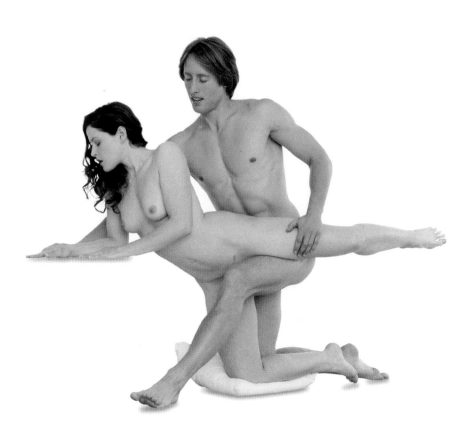

BEST FOR: beautifully choreographed sex
HITS THE SPOT FOR: coming gracefully
HOT TIP: do it to classical music

111 Pelvic exam

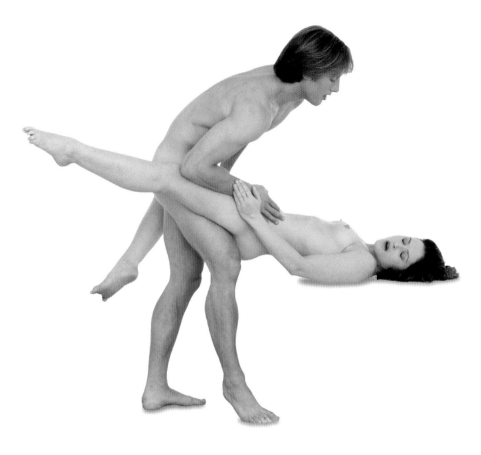

BEST FOR: men who know their way around
HITS THE SPOT FOR: "checking" that all her bits are in good working order
HOT TIP: pretend not to be aroused—until you penetrate her that is

Enchanted moment **112** _____

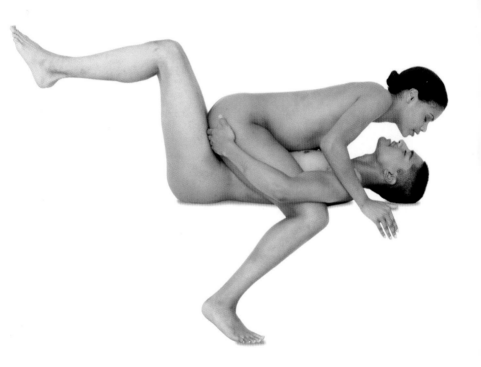

BEST FOR: when he's super-hard and she's super-wet _____
HITS THE SPOT FOR: experiencing the heady rush of those first few seconds
HOT TIP: stay perfectly still—don't even move an eyelash

113 Arms race

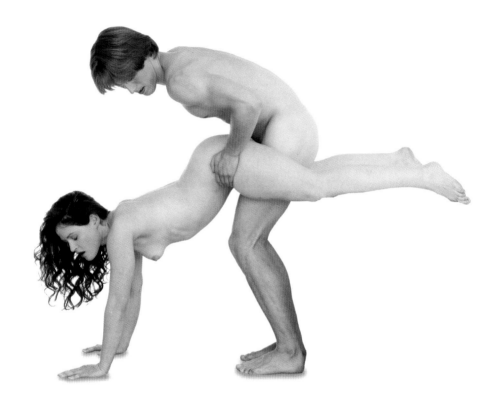

BEST FOR: you-better-make-this-quick sex
HITS THE SPOT FOR: quivering limbs and eye-popping sensations
HOT TIP: end up on the floor with him on top

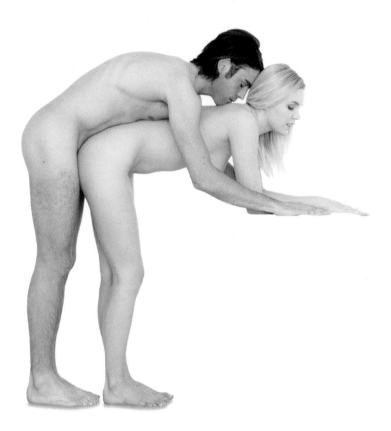

BEST FOR: sex while gripping the edge of the bathtub

HITS THE SPOT FOR: a saucy surprise—will it be anal or vaginal?

HOT TIP: don't follow anal sex with vaginal; the other way around is fine

115 Jet ski

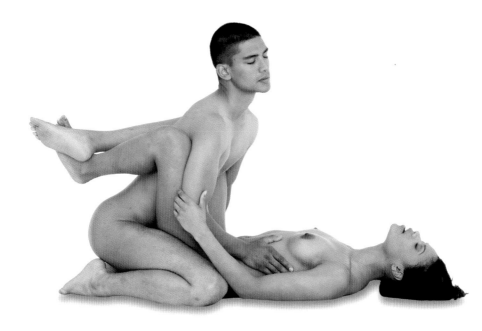

BEST FOR: quick and nimble sex
HITS THE SPOT FOR: fast, darting penis strokes
HOT TIP: if the height's not right, just add a couple of pillows underneath her

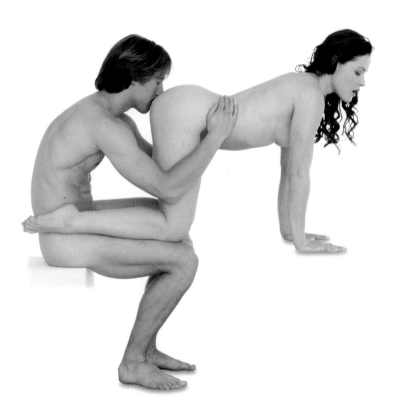

BEST FOR: when you want to explore alternative territory

HITS THE SPOT FOR: intimate kisses and licks that will turn her to liquid

HOT TIP: gently nip and nibble her cheeks

117 Keep it down

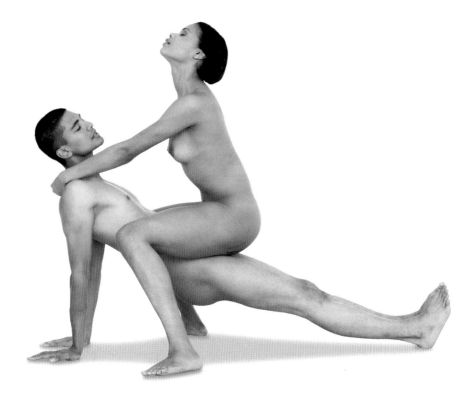

BEST FOR: sex when you mustn't be overheard
HITS THE SPOT FOR: not sounding like you're coming through the ceiling
HOT TIP: girls — clamp your hand over his mouth if he gets noisy

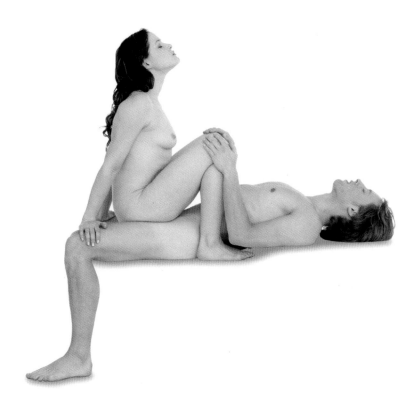

BEST FOR: when she's horny and needs to jump him

HITS THE SPOT FOR: fast back-and-forth clitoral stimulation

HOT TIP: guys—know when the hotspots are in her cycle. Be ready...

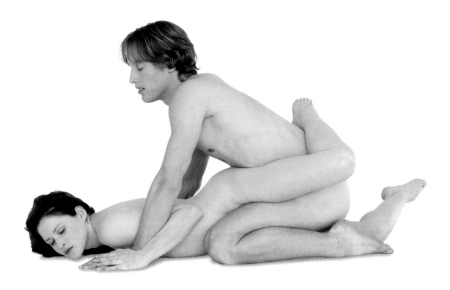

BEST FOR: sex with wave-like vaginal orgasms
HITS THE SPOT FOR: angling his penis so it makes a direct hit on her G-spot
HOT TIP: if G-spot pressure makes you want to pee, work through it

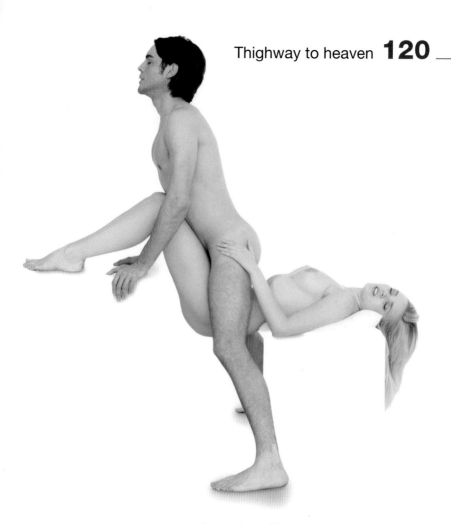

BEST FOR: femoral sex (thrusting between her thighs)
HITS THE SPOT FOR: a delectable penis massage between two soft surfaces
HOT TIP: coat yourselves in oil for the maximum in sensual slipperiness

121 The invisible seat

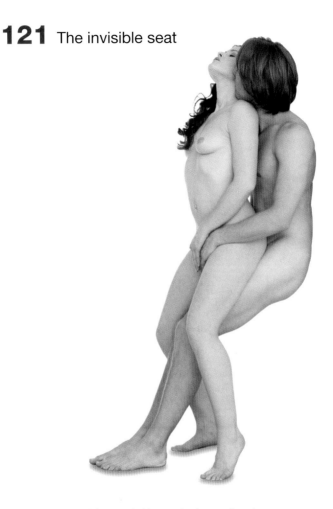

BEST FOR: an outdoor quickie against a wall or tree
HITS THE SPOT FOR: dignity if you're discovered—stand up and act natural
HOT TIP: guys—press yourself into that wall for support

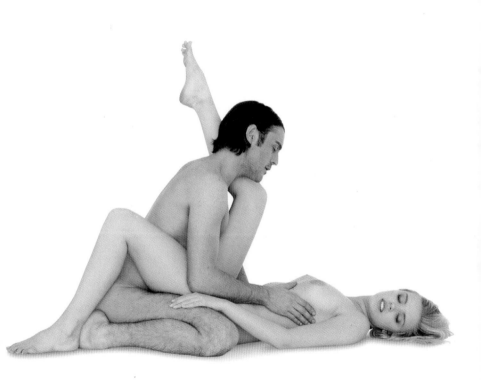

BEST FOR: long winter evenings
HITS THE SPOT FOR: oiled palms caressing each other's body
HOT TIP: purr, moan, sigh, and gasp

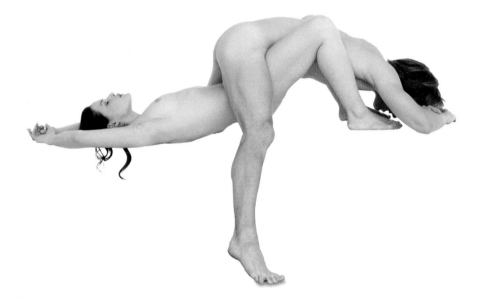

BEST FOR: supple-bodied lovers

HITS THE SPOT FOR: her having her toes kissed, licked, and nuzzled

HOT TIP: guys—try practicing your toe-job skills in a simpler position first

Halfway house 124 ____

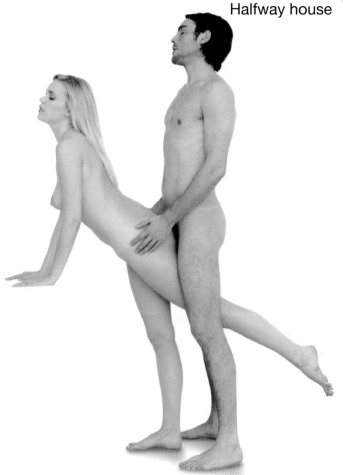

BEST FOR: a cheeky anal turn-on
HITS THE SPOT FOR: pressing his penis between her cheeks
HOT TIP: try this if you're an anal-sex novice

125 Rock-a-bye-baby

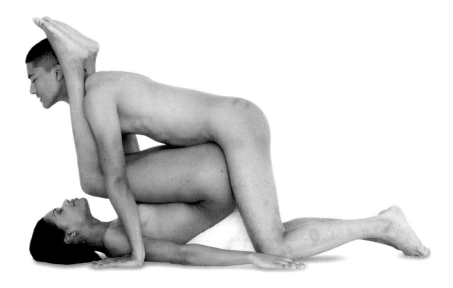

BEST FOR: when you have to have it right now
HITS THE SPOT FOR: the deepest possible penetration
HOT TIP: larger penises—move with caution

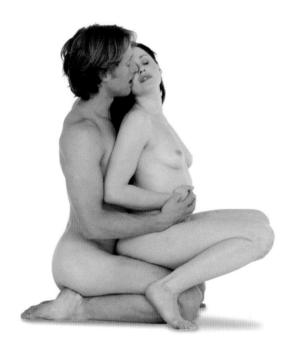

BEST FOR: very late pregnancy, when she's about to drop
HITS THE SPOT FOR: loving intimacy during the last few days
HOT TIP: it's also a good labor position (just not with him inside her)

127 The launch pad

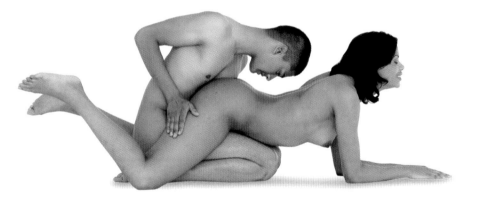

BEST FOR: when you're firing on all cylinders
HITS THE SPOT FOR: jet-propelled orgasms
HOT TIP: give an extra boost by sucking hard on her buttocks

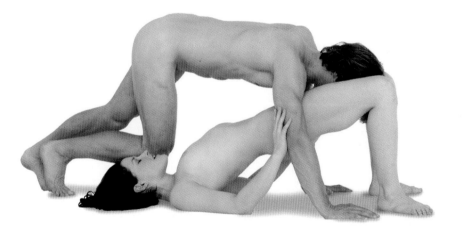

BEST FOR: couples who love doctor/patient games
HITS THE SPOT FOR: uninhibited playfulness
HOT TIP: firmly instruct her to "open her legs a little wider"

129 Front drape

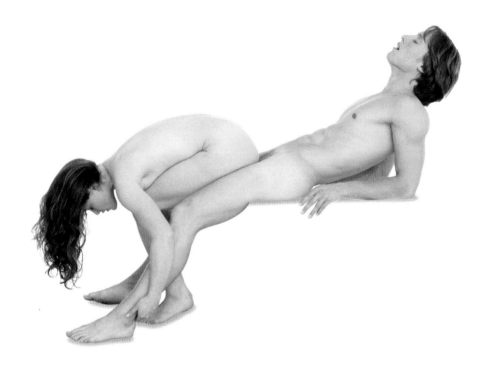

BEST FOR: when she's dropped something on the floor
HITS THE SPOT FOR: tugging his penis toward his feet
HOT TIP: girls—give him a foot rub while you're down there

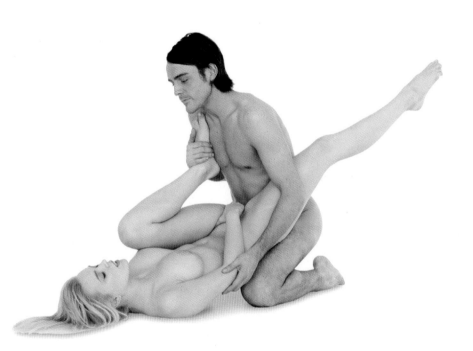

BEST FOR: girls who like a penis-plus-hand combo
HITS THE SPOT FOR: getting off on each other's arousal
HOT TIP: see if you can come at the same time

131 The camel

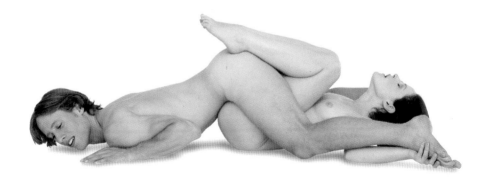

BEST FOR: when you want a change from face-to-face humping
HITS THE SPOT FOR: a cheeky massage from her heels
HOT TIP: don't say: "one hump or two?"

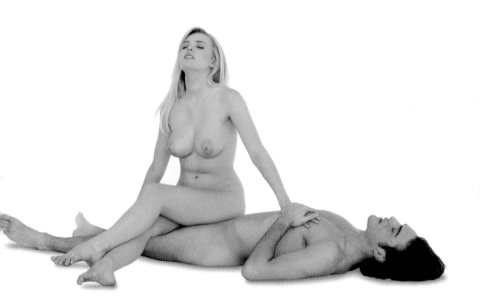

BEST FOR: sedate love when you're not itching to move
HITS THE SPOT FOR: him feeling deeply enclosed
HOT TIP: his penis is at an unusual angle, so no sudden movements

133 The swan dive

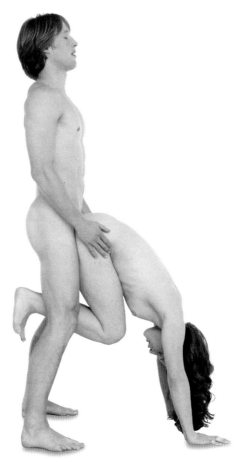

BEST FOR: when you're bored with the missionary position
HITS THE SPOT FOR: pure titillation for him
HOT TIP: don't suggest it if she's in bed with a head cold

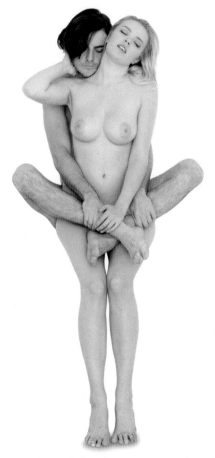

BEST FOR: when you're so intimate you can read each other's mind

HITS THE SPOT FOR: being up close and personal

HOT TIP: feel the loving energy flow between you

135 The love seat

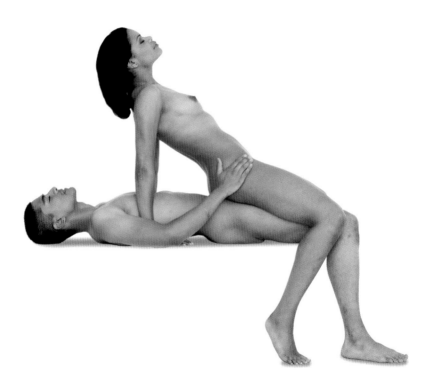

BEST FOR: when he doesn't want hard and fast thrusting
HITS THE SPOT FOR: making him last longer
HOT TIP: finish up in a more dynamic standing position

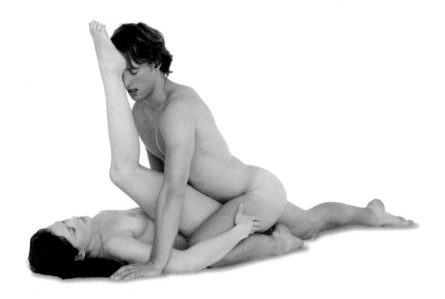

BEST FOR: when she wants a thigh work-out
HITS THE SPOT FOR: bringing him to heel
HOT TIP: if you haven't been to the gym in a while, put your foot on his chest

137 See you in the morning

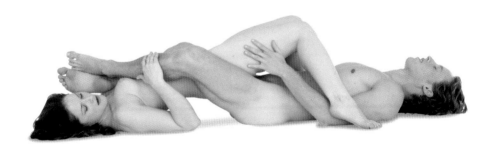

BEST FOR: we're-nearly-asleep-but-let's-do-it-anyway sex
HITS THE SPOT FOR: waking up and thinking: "how did I get here?"
HOT TIP: put a pillow at both ends of the bed

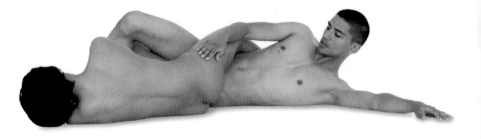

BEST FOR: sex on the floor
HITS THE SPOT FOR: a warm glow of relaxed sensuality
HOT TIP: let him do the moving

139 School's out

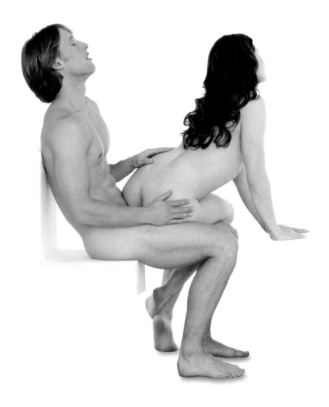

BEST FOR: when the kids are due home any second
HITS THE SPOT FOR: the efficiency of sex on borrowed time
HOT TIP: put a lock on your bedroom door

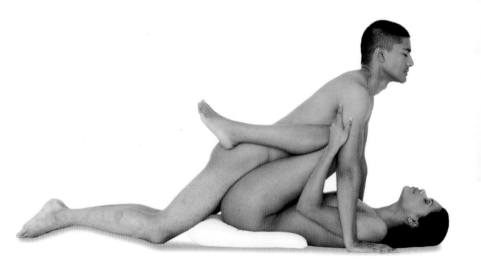

BEST FOR: the less well endowed man

HITS THE SPOT FOR: making her vagina shorter to maximize sensation

HOT TIP: the all-important cushion will help you plumb her depths

141 The grand finale

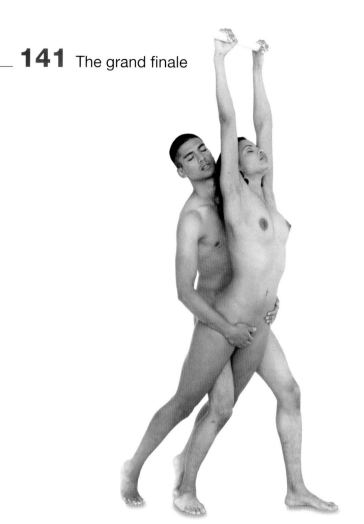

BEST FOR: those who enjoy graceful rear-entry
HITS THE SPOT FOR: head-to-toe tingles
HOT TIP: she needs to get into position first

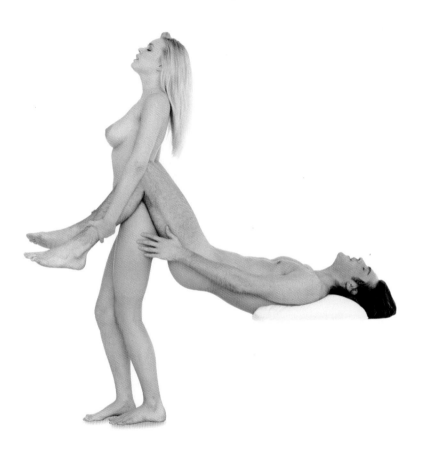

BEST FOR: when she's gotta have it and he's fallen asleep
HITS THE SPOT FOR: the naughtiness of dragging him off the bed
HOT TIP: don't expect him to then deliver a first-class performance

143 Bubbling love

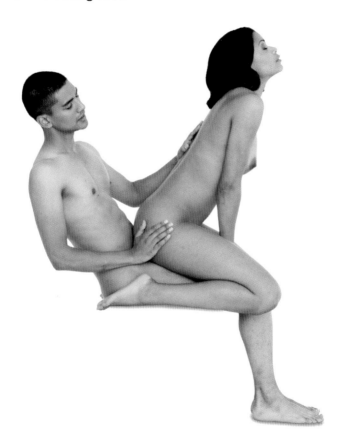

BEST FOR: getting jiggy in a jacuzzi
HITS THE SPOT FOR: tingles and tremors to make you moan
HOT TIP: position your favorite erogenous zone over a jet of bubbles

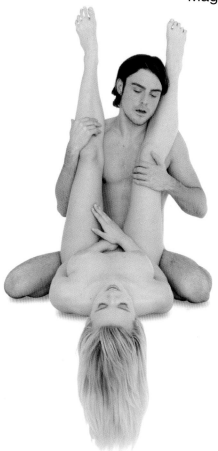

BEST FOR: anyone, anytime, anywhere
HITS THE SPOT FOR: being a one-stop cure for sexual frustration
HOT TIP: look into each other's eyes when you climax

145 No-fuss thrust

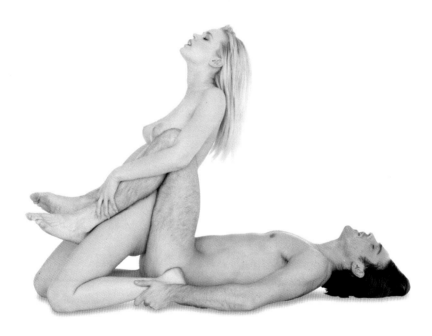

BEST FOR: pelvis pushers
HITS THE SPOT FOR: her staying still while he pumps up and down
HOT TIP: guys—wedge your heel next to her clitoris

Arm wrestle **146**

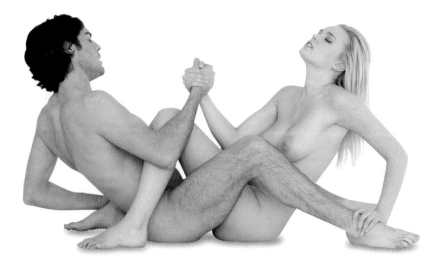

BEST FOR: when you've got a bone to pick with each other

HITS THE SPOT FOR: settling old scores by getting down and dirty

HOT TIP: ignore the advice about never going to bed while arguing

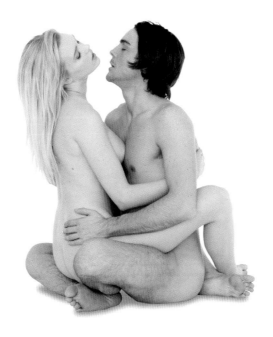

BEST FOR: tantric sex trainees
HITS THE SPOT FOR: getting connected—in mind, body, and spirit
HOT TIP: "can I slide my lingam into your yoni?"

Corner piece **148**

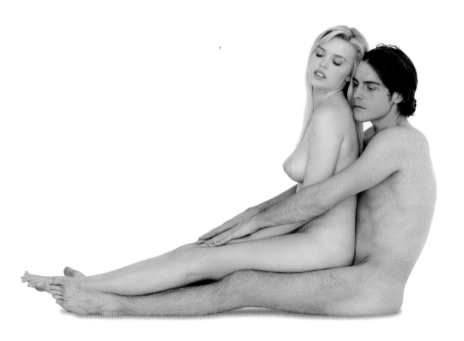

BEST FOR: when there's a handy wall to lean against
HITS THE SPOT FOR: being turned on and tuned in to each other
HOT TIP: guide his hand on your clitoris

149 I'll raise you

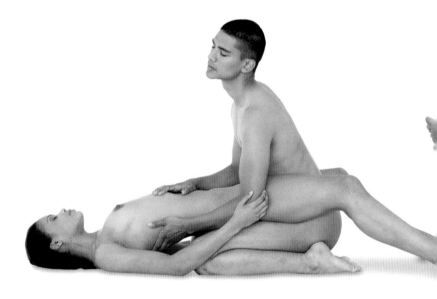

BEST FOR: when you want slow, considered sex
HITS THE SPOT FOR: the sensual bliss of a perfect fit
HOT TIP: girls — caress him with a vaginal squeeze

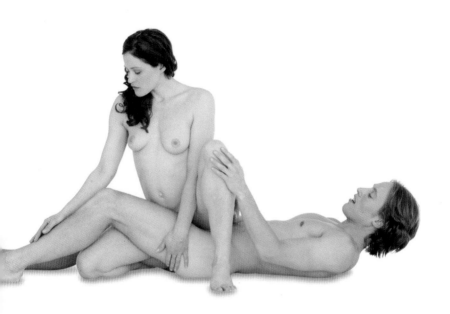

BEST FOR: shy lovers who like doing it in the dark
HITS THE SPOT FOR: the joy of experimenting with zero inhibitions
HOT TIP: squat, bend, arch, twist, and contort. Guys, that means you too

151 Service station

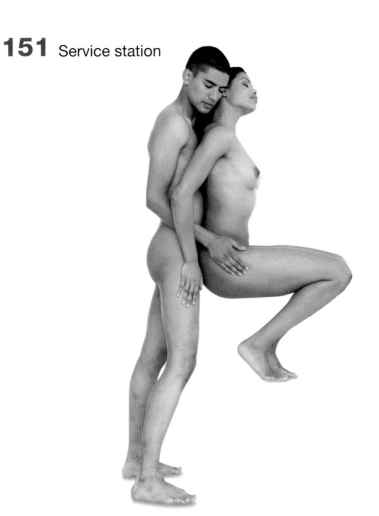

BEST FOR: giving her a personal valet service
HITS THE SPOT FOR: stroking her surfaces and lubricating her insides
HOT TIP: attend to her ear and neck—nibble, nuzzle, and lick

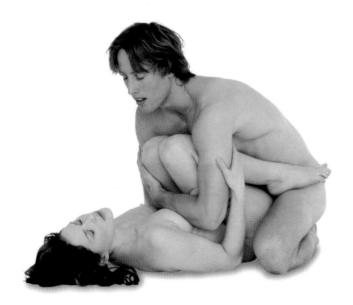

BEST FOR: men who tend to come quickly
HITS THE SPOT FOR: controlled thrusting that keeps a lid on his excitement
HOT TIP: if you think you're going to come, squeeze her knees tight

153 Lion king

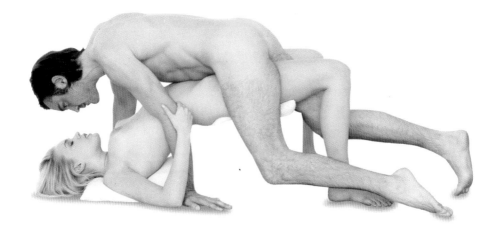

BEST FOR: hot predatory sex where he calls the shots
HITS THE SPOT FOR: dizzying pleasure and a rush of blood to her head
HOT TIP: if you don't normally talk dirty, do it now

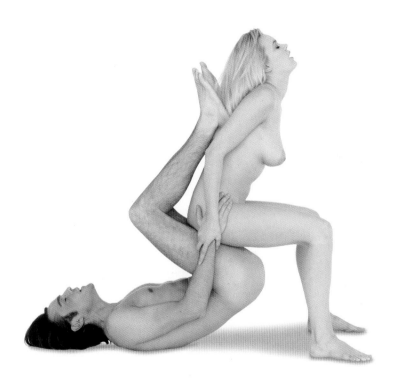

BEST FOR: when he's got a long yet floppy erection
HITS THE SPOT FOR: putting her in control
HOT TIP: girls—slide a lubed finger inside him to massage his prostate

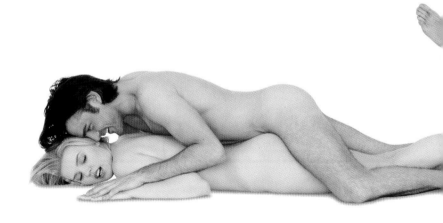

BEST FOR: when she's had a turn on top and now it's his turn
HITS THE SPOT FOR: being part of a long sexy sequence
HOT TIP: after this one, both get up on your hands and knees

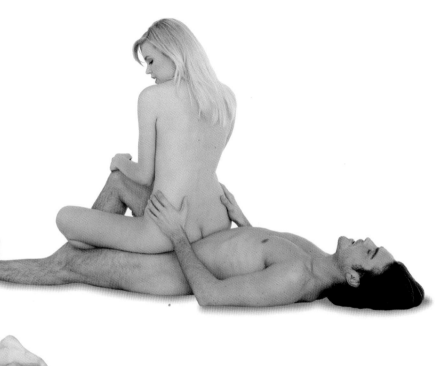

BEST FOR: when you're giving each other the silent treatment

HITS THE SPOT FOR: reconnecting through sex

HOT TIP: remember—the wildest sex can happen after an argument

157 Come as you are

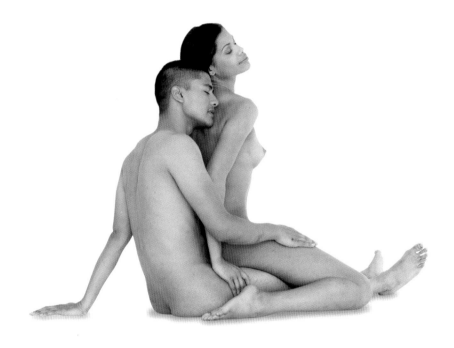

BEST FOR: when you've got something sexy to whisper
HITS THE SPOT FOR: hitting the high peaks of emotional arousal
HOT TIP: mid-sex compliments are always welcome—the bigger, the better

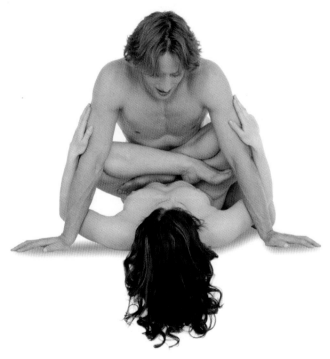

BEST FOR: Kama Sutra-style sex full of Eastern promise
HITS THE SPOT FOR: a fast climax in case she gets a charley horse first
HOT TIP: if she can't stretch to lotus pose, go cross-legged instead

159 Swimming lesson

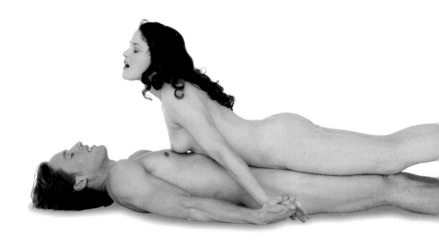

BEST FOR: practicing her stroke up and down his body
HITS THE SPOT FOR: a sensational tight pulling action on his penis
HOT TIP: sweat or oil will make for a smoother swim

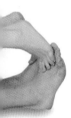

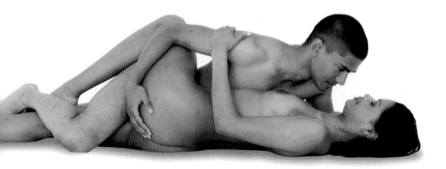

BEST FOR: make-up sex after an argument
HITS THE SPOT FOR: getting tenderly entwined
HOT TIP: take this moment to whisper "sorry"

161 Divine diver

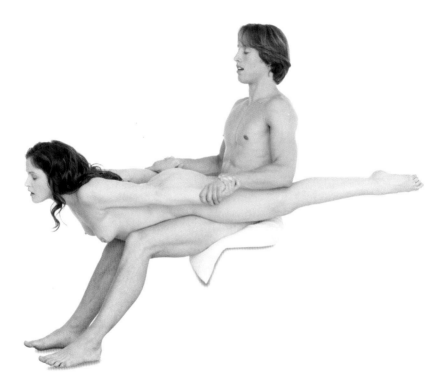

BEST FOR: couples with strong biceps
HITS THE SPOT FOR: making her feel deliciously taut
HOT TIP: if she wants the easy route, she can put her hands on the floor

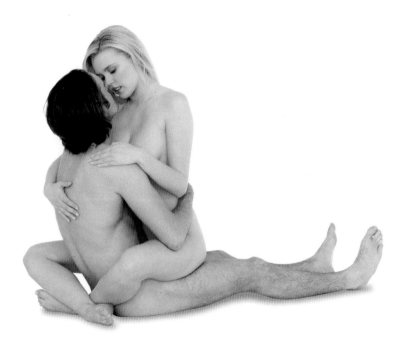

BEST FOR: cuddly snuggly sex
HITS THE SPOT FOR: expressing your tender side
HOT TIP: try it by candlelight

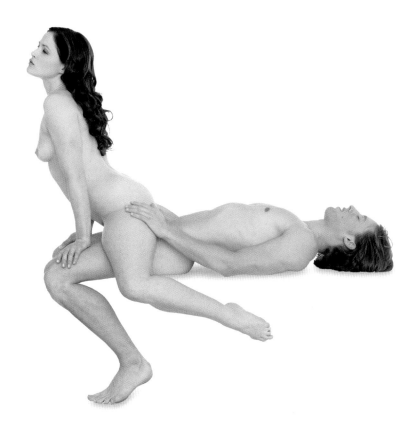

BEST FOR: when she wants to use him as a rocking horse
HITS THE SPOT FOR: satisfying pendulum-like movements on his penis
HOT TIP: for extra spice, add a fingertip vibrator

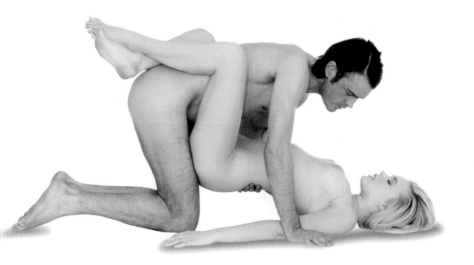

BEST FOR: when you've escaped upstairs at a party
HITS THE SPOT FOR: going at it hammer and tongs in the spare bedroom
HOT TIP: be good guests—leave no trace of your presence

165 Is that a gun in your purse?

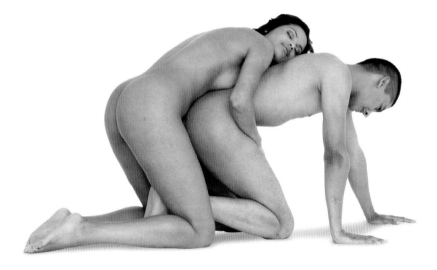

BEST FOR: girls who like to be boys
HITS THE SPOT FOR: kinky kicks from penetrating him with a strap-on dildo
HOT TIP: strap-ons not your style? Reach around and give him a hand job

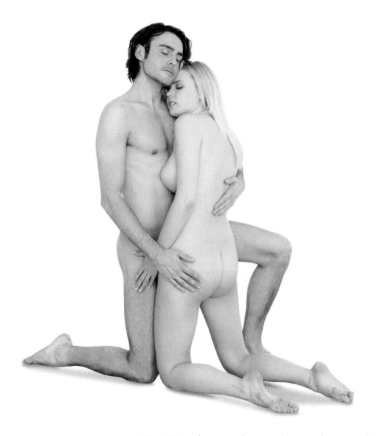

BEST FOR: when you're gearing up for round two
HITS THE SPOT FOR: between-sex cuddling while your genitals take a break
HOT TIP: fantasize about what's coming next

167 Push me, pull me

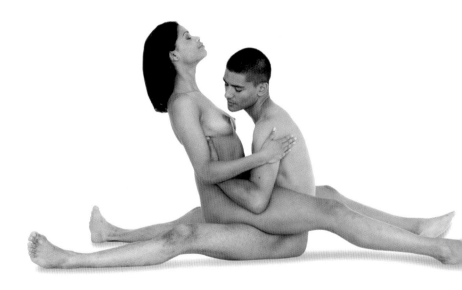

BEST FOR: when he's got a rock-like erection
HITS THE SPOT FOR: the luscious sensations of sliding on and off
HOT TIP: use lots of lube so you can slip against each other

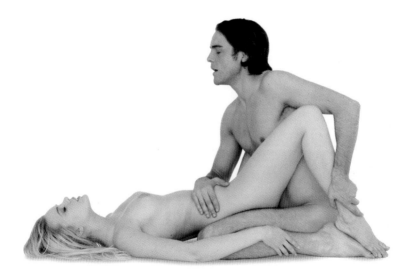

BEST FOR: an erotic reunion with an old lover
HITS THE SPOT FOR: swooning submission to his manly dominance
HOT TIP: plant the soles of your feet on his—and push

169 Spice merchant

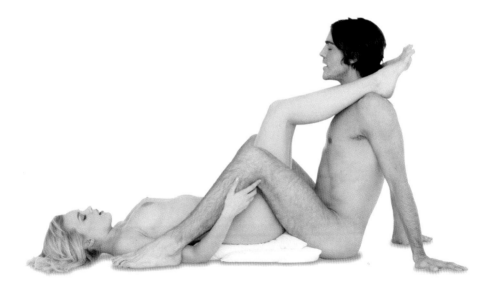

BEST FOR: when he wants to experiment
HITS THE SPOT FOR: him trying out a range of sex toys on her
HOT TIP: women—throw your inhibitions out the window. This is a treat

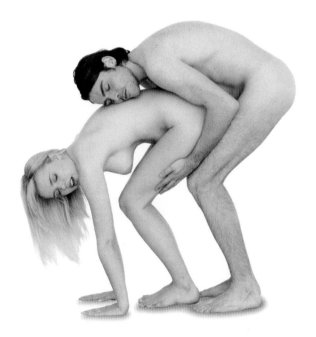

BEST FOR: late-night drunken sex
HITS THE SPOT FOR: fumbling, falling over, and not remembering the next day
HOT TIP: drink a glass of water before you go to bed

171 Passionfruit fizz

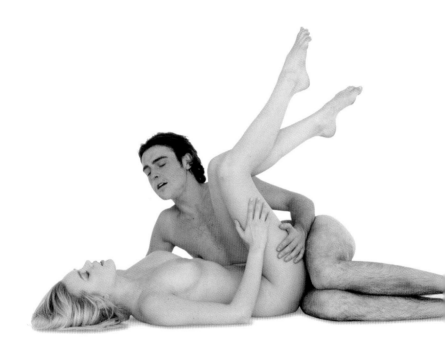

BEST FOR: when your arousal levels are sky high
HITS THE SPOT FOR: feasting on the sight of each other
HOT TIP: guys—use the quick, quick, slow approach to thrusting

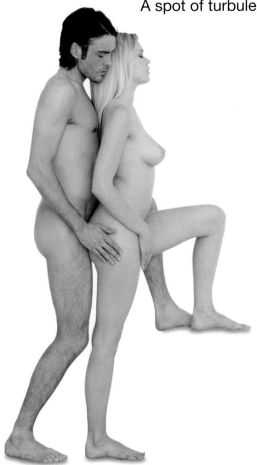

BEST FOR: lovers who want to join the mile-high club
HITS THE SPOT FOR: the thrill of a quickie in the toilet that you'll never forget
HOT TIP: return to your seats, fasten your seatbelts, look innocent

173 Chastity legs

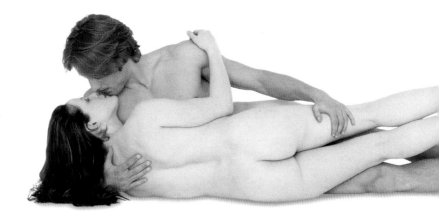

BEST FOR: when she's playing hard to get
HITS THE SPOT FOR: heavy petting and thigh-to-penis friction
HOT TIP: for proper penetration, she needs to open up a little

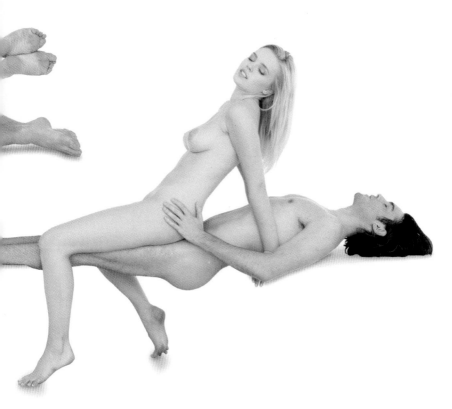

BEST FOR: when you need to hop on and off quickly
HITS THE SPOT FOR: that perfect feeling of full penetration
HOT TIP: if it feels structurally unsound, move the furniture closer together

175 I'm hooked on you

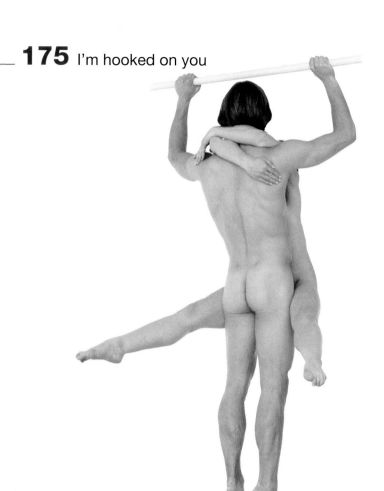

BEST FOR: sex that you can congratulate each other on
HITS THE SPOT FOR: getting a buzz from sex against the odds
HOT TIP: give yourself a break by wrapping your legs round his waist

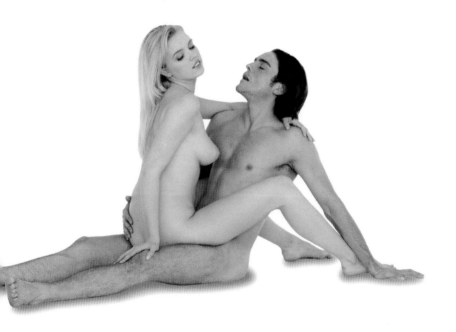

BEST FOR: lazy Sunday afternoons devoted to sex

HITS THE SPOT FOR: intimacy rather than intensity

HOT TIP: run your fingers down each other's back

177 Side straddle

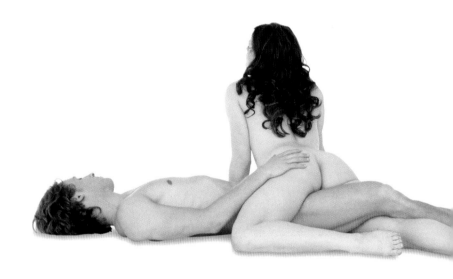

BEST FOR: when he wants easy access for spanking
HITS THE SPOT FOR: sexy undulating movements
HOT TIP: if you enjoy the spank, invest in a paddle

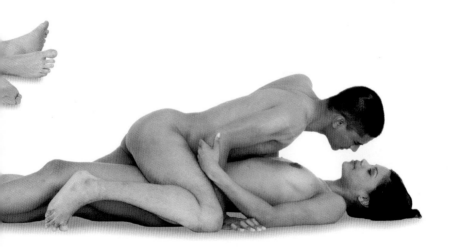

BEST FOR: the first time in bed with your new lover
HITS THE SPOT FOR: getting to know each other
HOT TIP: guys—take deep belly breaths if you think you're going to come

179 See-saw

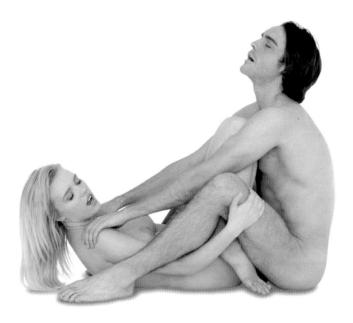

BEST FOR: calorie-burning sex
HITS THE SPOT FOR: her gripping him tightly with her vagina
HOT TIP: rock in a see-saw motion

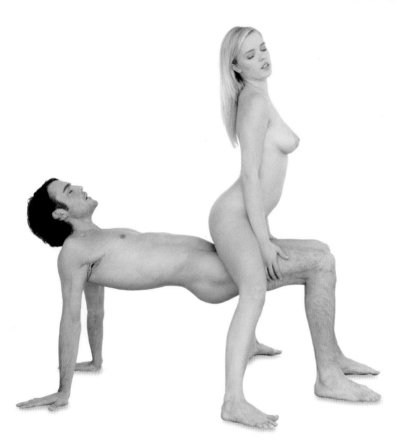

Mr. Chivalrous **180**

BEST FOR: sex in hostile terrain
HITS THE SPOT FOR: gentlemanly protection from pavement/tarmac/mud
HOT TIP: repay him with a sexual favor you know he'll love

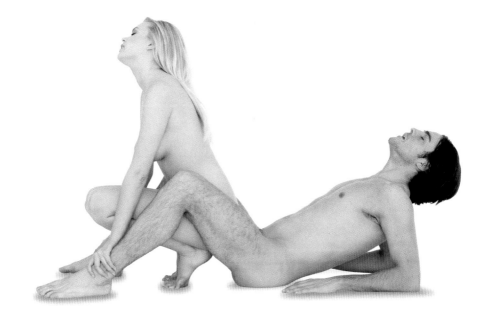

BEST FOR: when he's got some strong lead in his pencil
HITS THE SPOT FOR: the voluptuous sensation of withdrawing on every stroke
HOT TIP: if he responds like a piece of wilted lettuce, put this one on hold

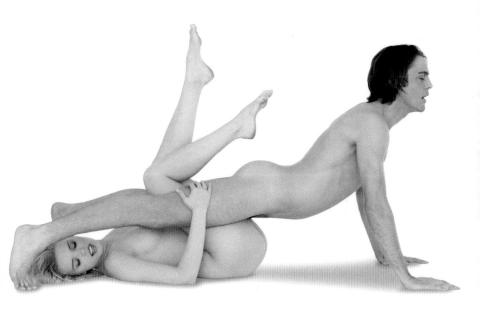

BEST FOR: super-gymnastic sex
HITS THE SPOT FOR: showing off your sexual versatility
HOT TIP: guys—if you need a well-earned break, rest on your forearms

183 Neck brace

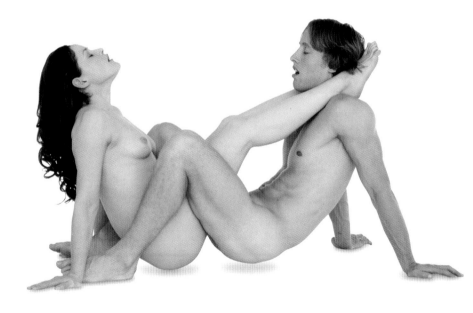

BEST FOR: when you don't want sex in the same old way
HITS THE SPOT FOR: some daring and creative eroticism
HOT TIP: be gentle—despite what they say, asphyxiation isn't erotic

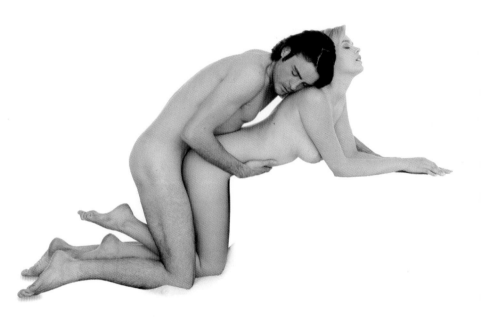

BEST FOR: rear penetration with comfort and grace

HITS THE SPOT FOR: snuggling your bodies together

HOT TIP: see yourself at your sexiest—do it in front of a mirror

185 I know what you did last night

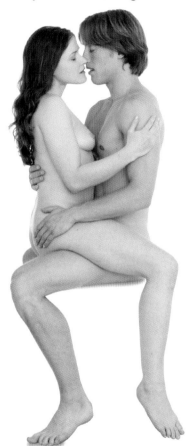

BEST FOR: sex on a swing
HITS THE SPOT FOR: putting a smile on your face the next day
HOT TIP: don't get arrested

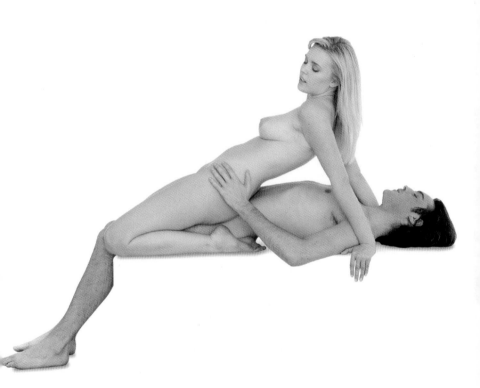

BEST FOR: snaky hip movers
HITS THE SPOT FOR: making her feel gorgeous, and him feel on fire
HOT TIP: women—alternate between fast flicks and super-slow ripples

187 Pick-me-up

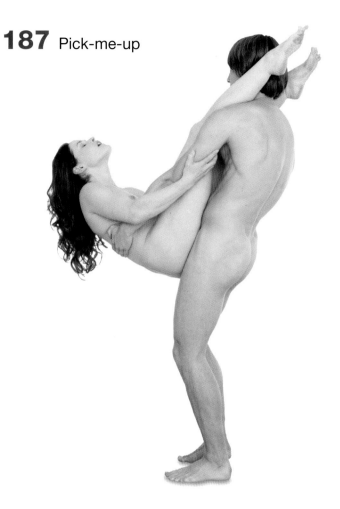

BEST FOR: the lightweight lady
HITS THE SPOT FOR: a sexy display of male muscle
HOT TIP: get into it from a lying-down position when she's on top

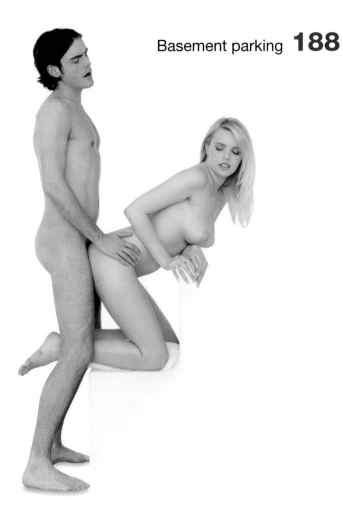

BEST FOR: lovers who enjoy navigating tight anal corners

HITS THE SPOT FOR: the joy of resting his penis in a compact space

HOT TIP: small cars are the easiest to park

189 Come sit at my table

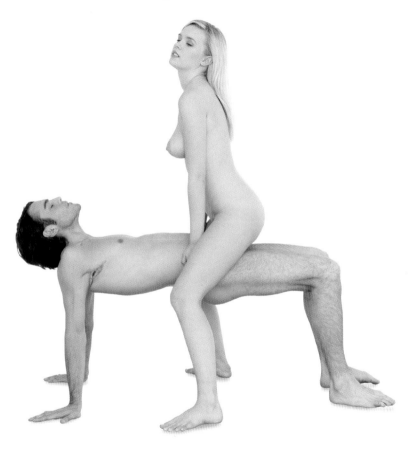

BEST FOR: guys with strong limbs and strong erections
HITS THE SPOT FOR: the sheer excitement of straddle-and-go sex
HOT TIP: girls, pretend you're on a horse — now ride it

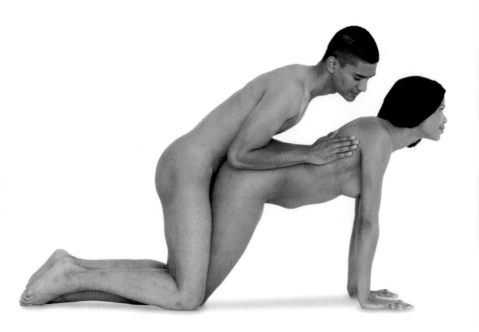

BEST FOR: when time is short
HITS THE SPOT FOR: being gentler than The deep dog (see 89)
HOT TIP: she can hold a vibrator against her clitoris for extra buzz

191 That lovin' feeling

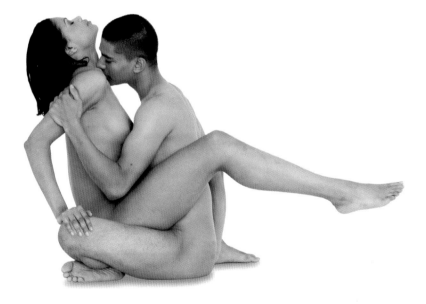

BEST FOR: when you want to rediscover lost intimacy
HITS THE SPOT FOR: feeling warm and fuzzy inside again
HOT TIP: pepper the whole day with sultry kisses and sexy compliments

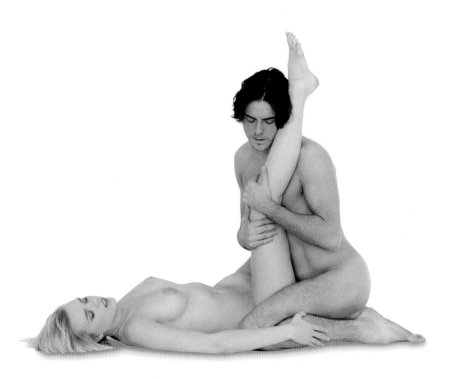

BEST FOR: when she's got her sexiest stockings on
HITS THE SPOT FOR: making him explode with desire
HOT TIP: ladies—choose your favorite sexy track and do a surprise strip

193 Room with a view

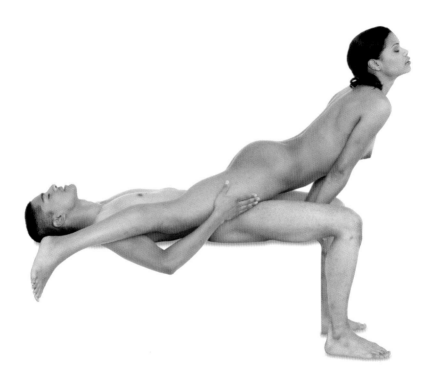

BEST FOR: sex while she looks out the window
HITS THE SPOT FOR: making sure her roommate isn't coming home
HOT TIP: guys—raise your head for your very own private view

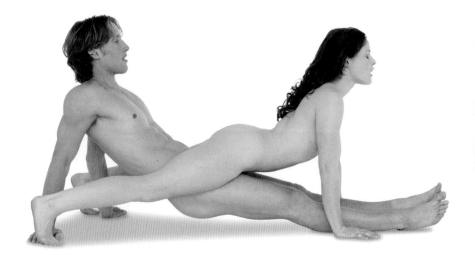

BEST FOR: couples who like to work out together
HITS THE SPOT FOR: pretending that sex is just a way of keeping fit
HOT TIP: launch your own range of sexercise DVDs

195 One-legged love

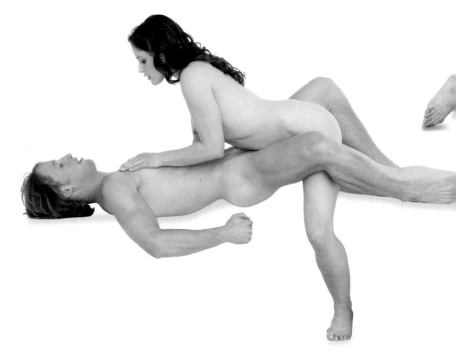

BEST FOR: lovers who like to maneuver
HITS THE SPOT FOR: the fun of erotic exploration
HOT TIP: move the furniture until it all comes together

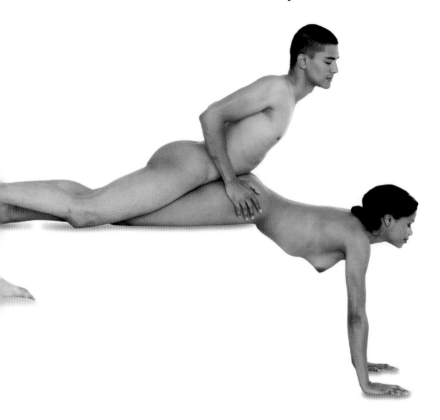

BEST FOR: strong-armed girls
HITS THE SPOT FOR: him sinking deeply into her
HOT TIP: if it's tricky, try slithering onto the floor while you're still joined

197 The empress

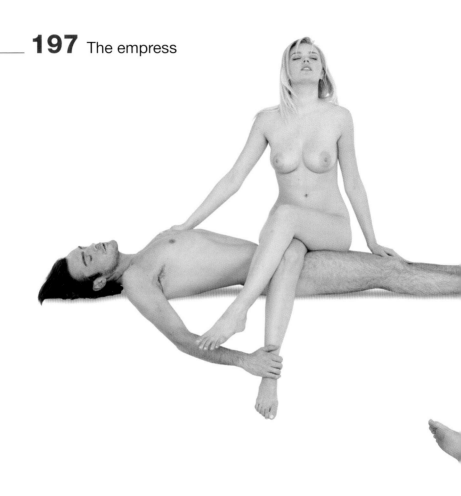

BEST FOR: casual climb-on sex
HITS THE SPOT FOR: an orgasm that he can barely suppress
HOT TIP: do it S-L-O-W

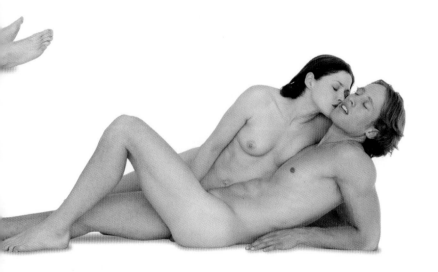

BEST FOR: when you've been at it all night
HITS THE SPOT FOR: wringing out that final erection
HOT TIP: once he's at least semi-erect, pop a cock ring on him

199 Legs wide open

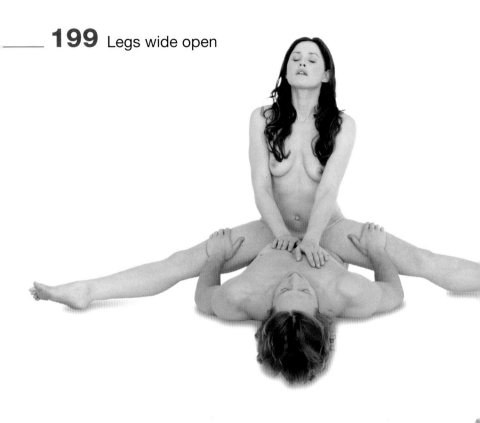

BEST FOR: trying-out-her-new-vibrator sex
HITS THE SPOT FOR: penetration plus vibes means double the pleasure
HOT TIP: get a contoured "woman-shaped" vibrator and pop it between you

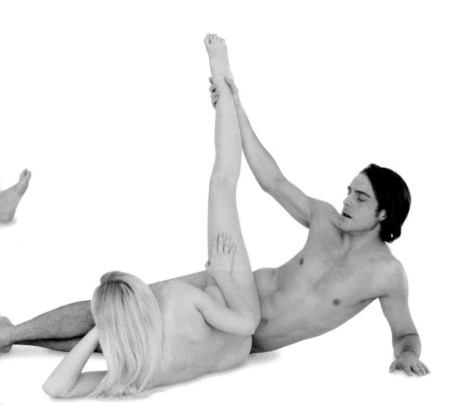

BEST FOR: experimental sex with a new lover
HITS THE SPOT FOR: discovering what's hot and what's not
HOT TIP: afterwards, play: "I liked it best when you…"

201 Lying down on the job

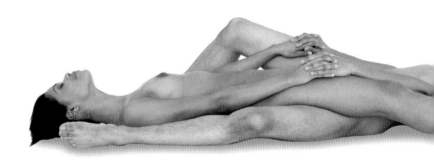

BEST FOR: when one of you ate garlic for dinner
HITS THE SPOT FOR: guaranteed by-hand orgasm (for her)
HOT TIP: to enhance this position, add a vibrator

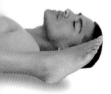

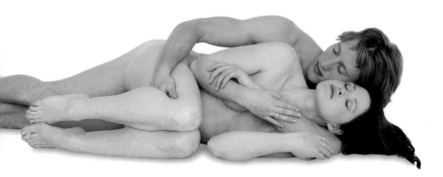

BEST FOR: preparing to lose your anal virginity
HITS THE SPOT FOR: prior fingertip exploration
HOT TIP: there's no such thing as too much lube

203 Adult education

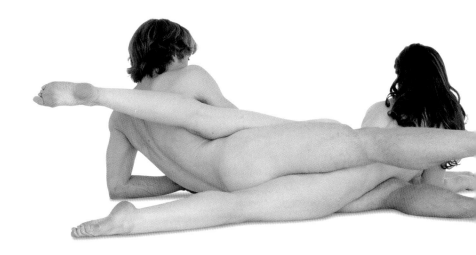

BEST FOR: exploring the realms of possibility
HITS THE SPOT FOR: having a laugh
HOT TIP: make it your mission to reinvent the Kama Sutra

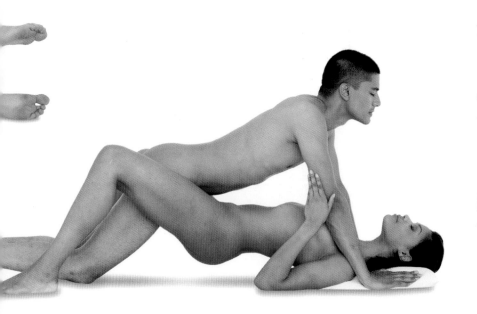

BEST FOR: your opening move to a day in bed
HITS THE SPOT FOR: non-stop joyous gyrating
HOT TIP: eat a sustaining energy snack afterward

205 The love object

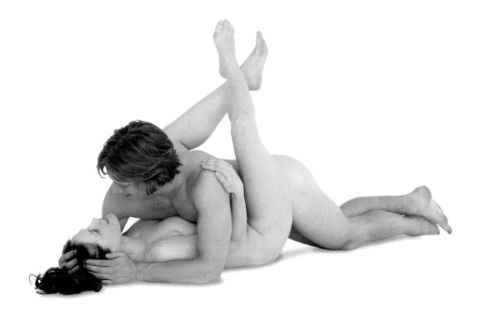

BEST FOR: hot honeymoon sex
HITS THE SPOT FOR: a sumptuous blend of lust, love, and sensuality
HOT TIP: don't get out of bed for days

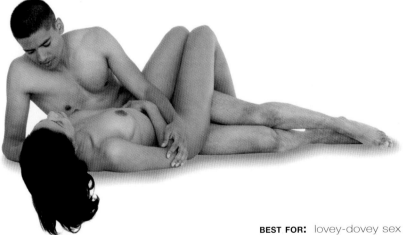

BEST FOR: lovey-dovey sex
HITS THE SPOT FOR: deep yet comfortable penetration
HOT TIP: a good one if she's heavily pregnant

207 The workout

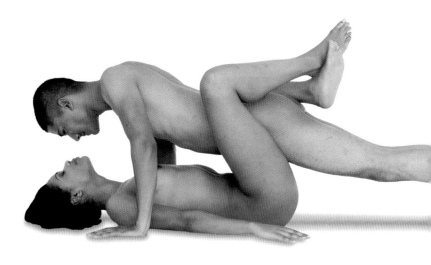

BEST FOR: when he wants to show off his biceps
HITS THE SPOT FOR: fast, precision pounding
HOT TIP: cheat by dropping your knees to the floor

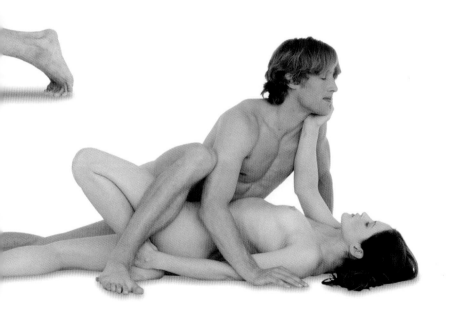

BEST FOR: moments of passionate urgency
HITS THE SPOT FOR: enjoying some fast-paced entwinement
HOT TIP: keep your bodies taut and tense until the end

209 Bow and arrow

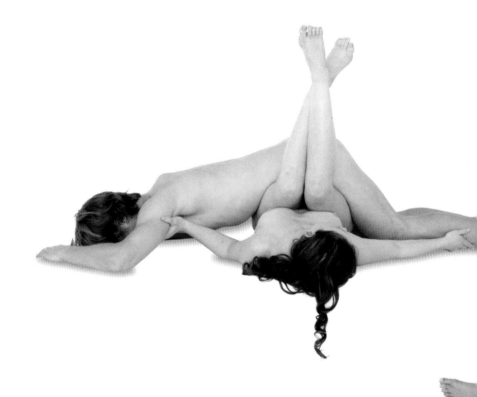

BEST FOR: artistic sex to impress an audience
HITS THE SPOT FOR: feeling sleek and gorgeous
HOT TIP: so what if you haven't got an audience? Fantasize

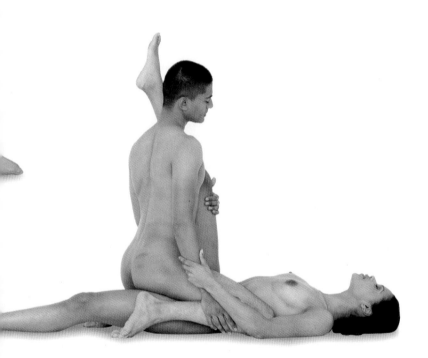

BEST FOR: when he wants to hold but not crowd her
HITS THE SPOT FOR: giving him a solid pillar to hold onto
HOT TIP: walk your fingertips from her calf to her thigh

211 The gameplan

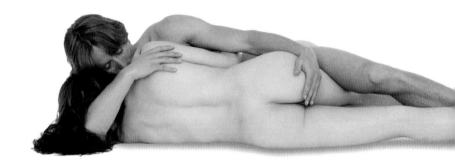

BEST FOR: a mid-sex break if he's going to climax too soon
HITS THE SPOT FOR: turning arousal down a notch
HOT TIP: take the opportunity for some tongue twining

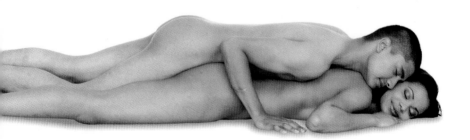

BEST FOR: sex on a twin bed
HITS THE SPOT FOR: rocking and rolling
HOT TIP: cuddle and gyrate at the same time

213 Hayloft

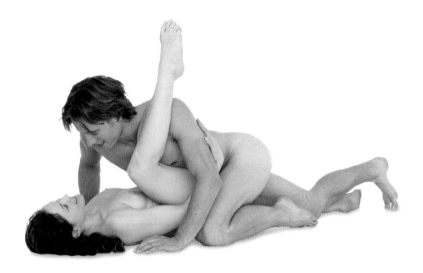

BEST FOR: clandestine meetings
HITS THE SPOT FOR: tantalizing closeness—you can almost kiss but not quite
HOT TIP: kiss your way from her toe to her thigh—then enter

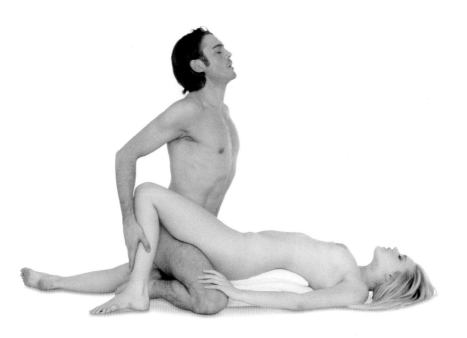

BEST FOR: luxurious sex on a silk-sheeted bed
HITS THE SPOT FOR: smooth, velvety sensations
HOT TIP: shave off all your pubes (yes, both of you) for the silkiest friction

215 Do the twist

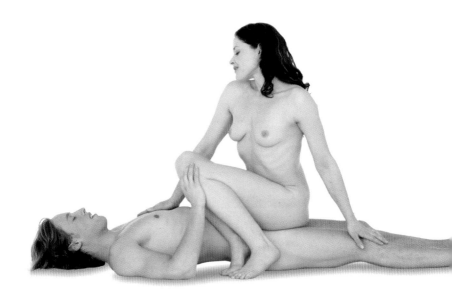

BEST FOR: twisting from a face-to-face position to a rear-entry position
HITS THE SPOT FOR: the fun of sexperimentation
HOT TIP: try twisting the other way too

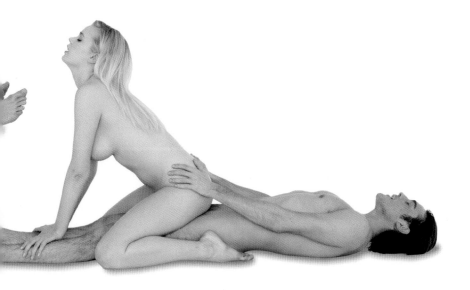

BEST FOR: fat days and bad hair days ————
HITS THE SPOT FOR: boosting your confidence when you're not at your best
HOT TIP: try it by candlelight

217 One lady driver

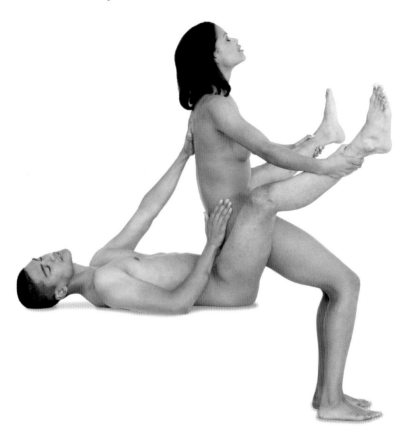

BEST FOR: role reversal—she's usually the one with her legs in the air
HITS THE SPOT FOR: the fun of some light-hearted boundary-breaking
HOT TIP: take role reversal to the next step; try cross-dressing

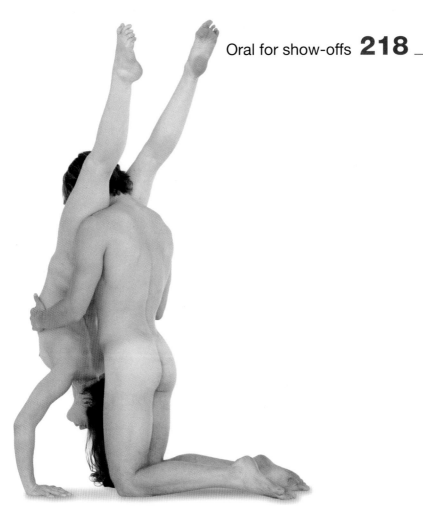

BEST FOR: professional sexperts ___
HITS THE SPOT FOR: stunning your friends at a sex party
HOT TIP: don't waste time nibbling her thighs, go straight for her hotspots

219 The gynecologist

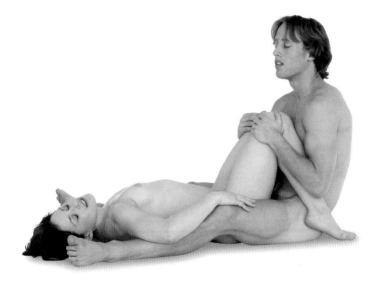

BEST FOR: when she's getting tired
HITS THE SPOT FOR: giving her a thorough internal exam
HOT TIP: use your hands as well as your penis

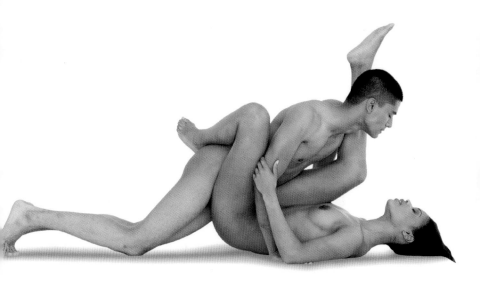

BEST FOR: going-with-the-flow sex
HITS THE SPOT FOR: feverish emotional and physical intensity
HOT TIP: do it on the floor so you can roll around to your heart's content

221 Intersection

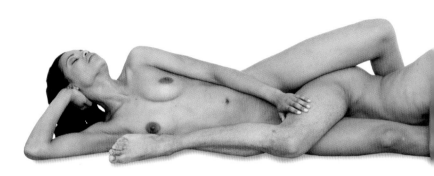

BEST FOR: those who like a challenge
HITS THE SPOT FOR: finding out how flexible his penis really is
HOT TIP: giggle if it goes wrong

The handyman **222**

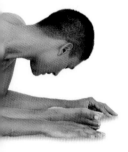

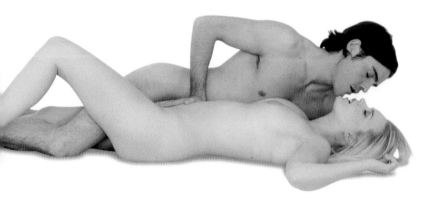

BEST FOR: when she's in need of his manual skills

HITS THE SPOT FOR: stroking, rubbing, sliding…and other tricks of the trade

HOT TIP: give her vagina and G-spot some creative handiwork too

223 Lip service

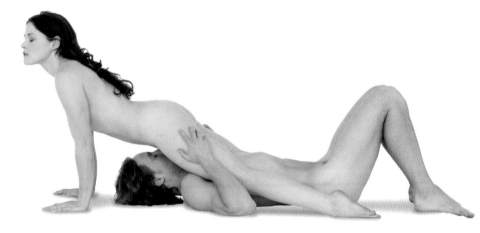

BEST FOR: the "lite" version of her sitting on his face
HITS THE SPOT FOR: irresistible tongue flicks on her love button
HOT TIP: if you can't hold the position, kneel with your knees by his ears

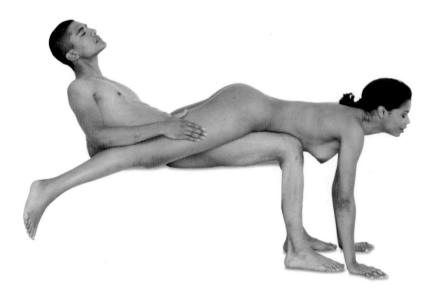

BEST FOR: when a beautiful bottom is his ultimate turn-on
HITS THE SPOT FOR: him feeling like he's being given a gift
HOT TIP: it's within your grasp—stroke it, spank it…gaze at it

225 The smooch dog

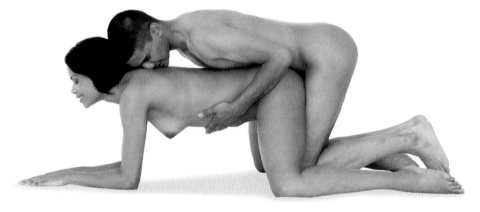

BEST FOR: a more intimate version of The deep dog (see 89)
HITS THE SPOT FOR: sexy nuzzling and whispering
HOT TIP: slide your palms along her front and give her nipples a tweak

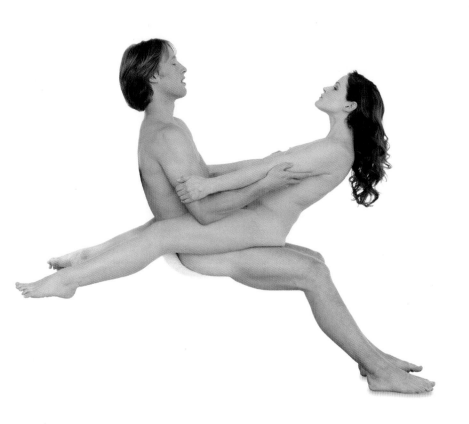

BEST FOR: when he wants to be ridden
HITS THE SPOT FOR: fast, fierce orgasms
HOT TIP: do it at the very peak of arousal

227 The wallflower

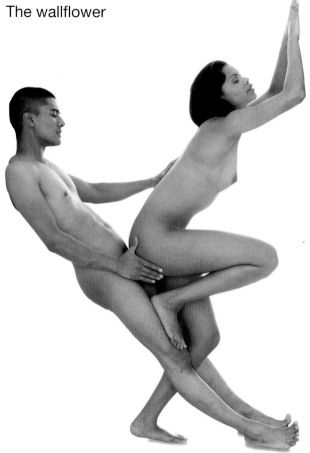

BEST FOR: lovers who aren't shy
HITS THE SPOT FOR: exquisite penetrate-to-the-core sensations
HOT TIP: gently cup your hands around her buttocks

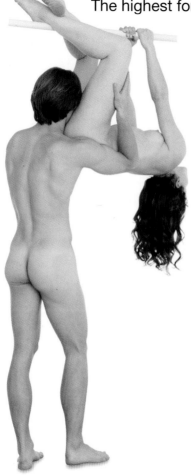

BEST FOR: cunnilingus connoisseurs who like variety
HITS THE SPOT FOR: dizzying heights of pleasure
HOT TIP: now's the time for a firm hand on her back

229 Driving Miss Daisy

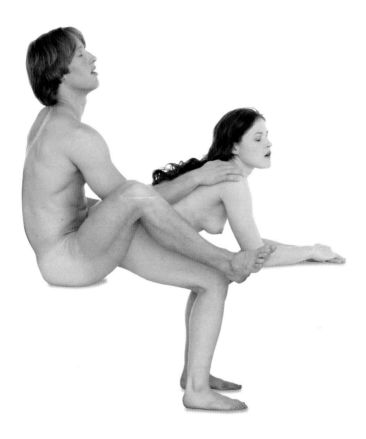

BEST FOR: when he likes using his penis to stroke her bits
HITS THE SPOT FOR: sending shivers up her spine
HOT TIP: caress her back with your hands—all the way from nape to anus

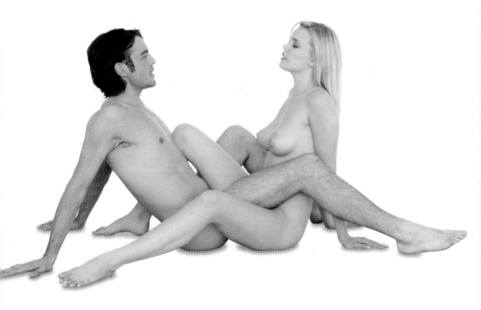

BEST FOR: sweet, fruity moments
HITS THE SPOT FOR: tickling both the taste buds and the sex buds
HOT TIP: feed strawberries to each other and drizzle each other with cream

231 The man trap

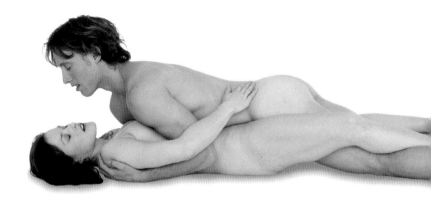

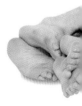

BEST FOR: sex with a hint of bondage
HITS THE SPOT FOR: pinning his legs in position with her feet
HOT TIP: girls—do it dressed in latex, and don't let him escape!

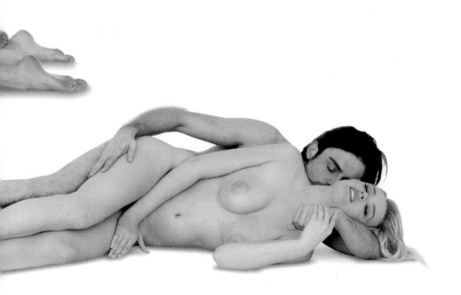

BEST FOR: half-asleep middle-of-the-night sex
HITS THE SPOT FOR: lazy yet tender loving
HOT TIP: murmur "g'night" before falling asleep in the same position

233 Are you serious?

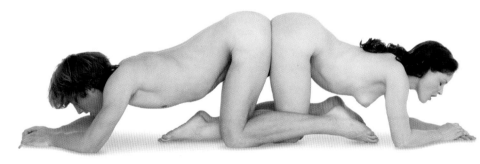

BEST FOR: sex-meets-sculpture
HITS THE SPOT FOR: cheek-to-cheek intimacy
HOT TIP: get someone to take a picture of you

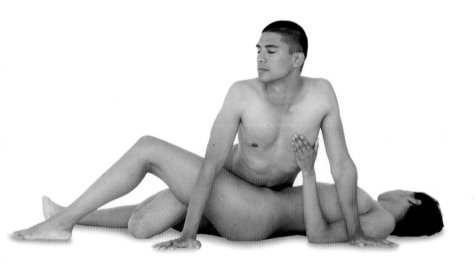

BEST FOR: those looking for a new angle
HITS THE SPOT FOR: finding vaginal pleasure zones she never knew she had
HOT TIP: swivel your body toward her head or her feet while still inside her

235 Scarlet harlot

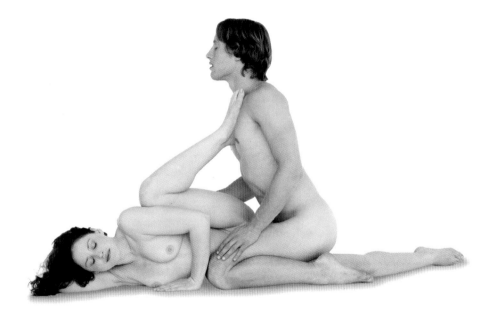

BEST FOR: masochistic boys—and the girls who whip them into shape
HITS THE SPOT FOR: acting like the stars of an X-rated movie
HOT TIP: bind his wrists and press your stilettoed heel into his chest

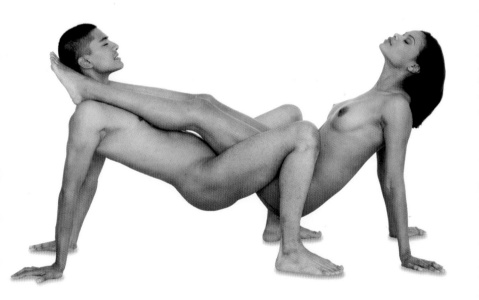

BEST FOR: couples who are competitive
HITS THE SPOT FOR: seeing who can hold the position longest
HOT TIP: make the loser a sex slave for the next hour

237 Cradle love

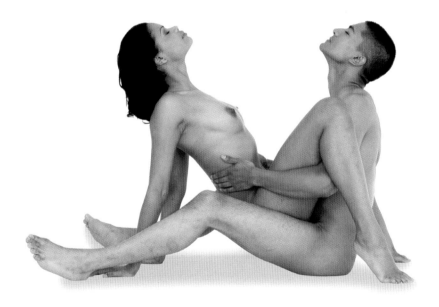

BEST FOR: stationary sex
HITS THE SPOT FOR: seeing eye-to-eye
HOT TIP: flex your penis inside her

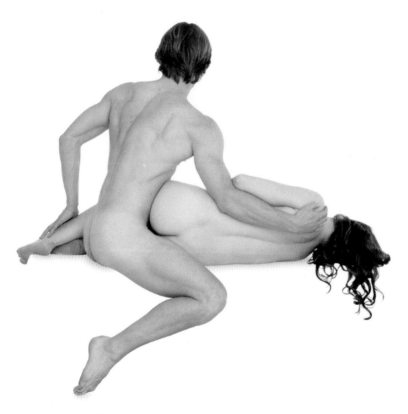

BEST FOR: gentle "medicinal" sex
HITS THE SPOT FOR: her playing a passive role
HOT TIP: make it part of a role play

239 Want to lie down?

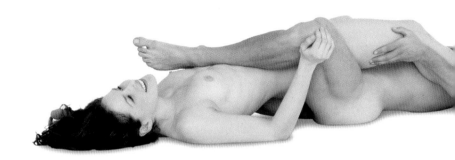

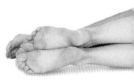

BEST FOR: when you can't decide who should go on top
HITS THE SPOT FOR: feelings of intimately joined togetherness
HOT TIP: up the romance factor—hold hands

Bedtime story **240**

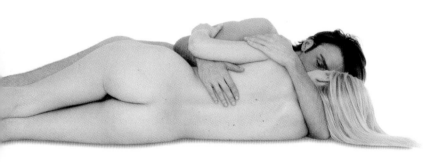

BEST FOR: when you want to whisper erotic tales between the sheets

HITS THE SPOT FOR: making the air crackle with sexual tension

HOT TIP: like all good stories, yours should end with a dramatic climax

241 The rabbit lift

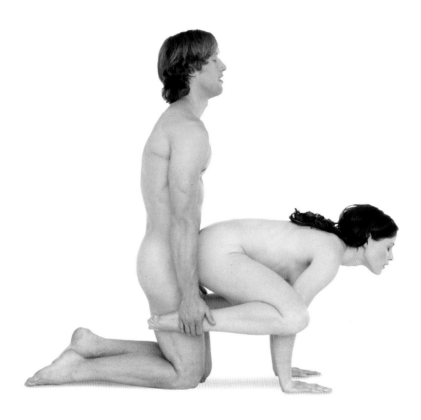

BEST FOR: sex on a firm piece of ground
HITS THE SPOT FOR: precarious thrills
HOT TIP: don't rely on her to do the moving

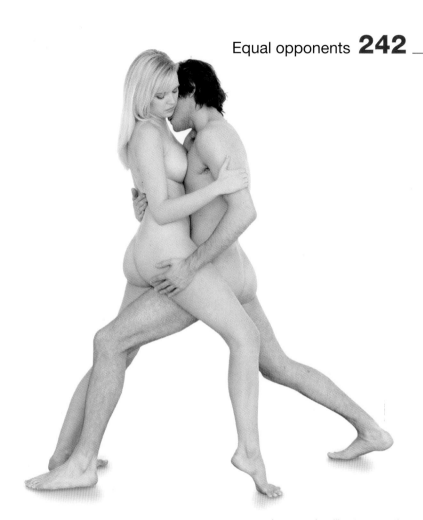

BEST FOR: lovers who like to wrestle

HITS THE SPOT FOR: the abandon of slamming your bodies into one another

HOT TIP: if penetration is tricky, she can hitch a ride on his thigh

243 The carnal couch

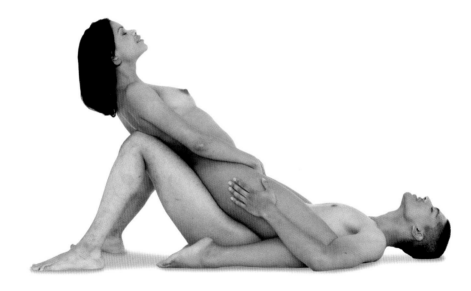

BEST FOR: sex on the couch instead of the bed
HITS THE SPOT FOR: comfortable sex that brings you close
HOT TIP: don't let sex become too familiar

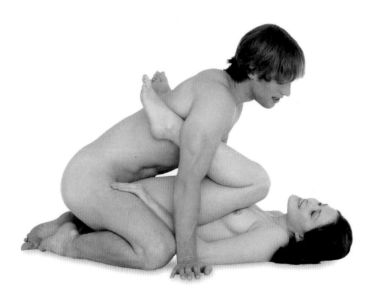

BEST FOR: sex in small spaces
HITS THE SPOT FOR: body-tingling deep penetration
HOT TIP: raise the game with a pile of cushions

245 The crouching tigress

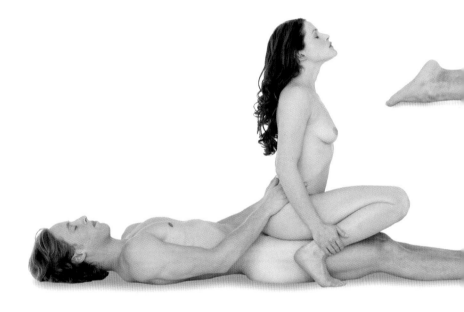

BEST FOR: when she's the boss in the relationship
HITS THE SPOT FOR: his view of her sexy bottom
HOT TIP: move your pelvis in small circles (like a miniature belly dance)

Half-pounder **246**

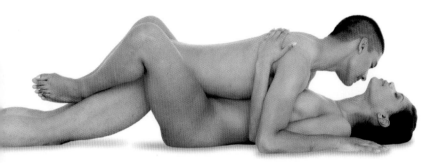

BEST FOR: when he wants to climax fast
HITS THE SPOT FOR: no-holds-barred thrusting
HOT TIP: the higher her knees, the deeper he can plunge

247 The flower press

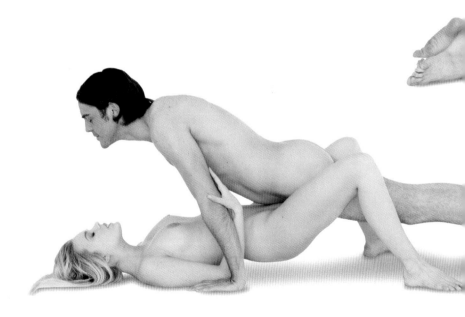

BEST FOR: men who can hold that push-up position
HITS THE SPOT FOR: sharing long, lustful looks
HOT TIP: girls—flick your hips up and down while he stays still

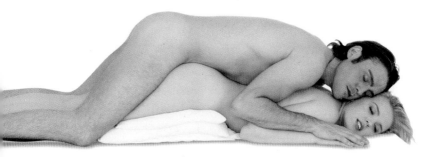

BEST FOR: the cozy variety of anal sex
HITS THE SPOT FOR: feeling very intimate, yet very, very naughty
HOT TIP: if you're adventurous, swap — she can take him with a strap-on

249 The swing

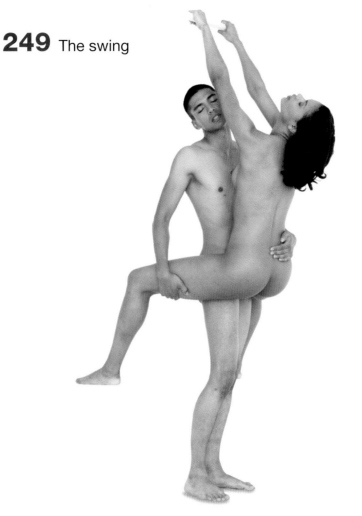

BEST FOR: adrenaline junkies
HITS THE SPOT FOR: lots of strong friction as she swings on and off his shaft
HOT TIP: guys—you'll need a firm footing

The saint **250** ___

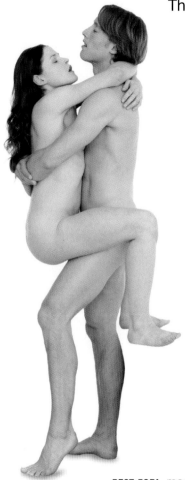

BEST FOR: moods of pure lechery ___
HITS THE SPOT FOR: sweeping her off her feet
HOT TIP: try it in a pool, it's easier

251 69—but not as you know it

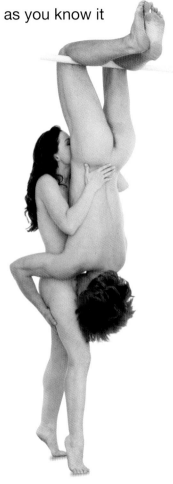

BEST FOR: when the horizontal equivalent brings on a yawn
HITS THE SPOT FOR: the thrill of performing a sexual party trick
HOT TIP: get your tongues moving fast—this won't be an all-nighter

Squat 'n' bounce **252**

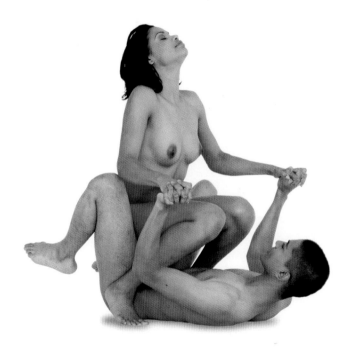

BEST FOR: girls with thighs of steel
HITS THE SPOT FOR: the thrill of her being in the driver's seat
HOT TIP: it's hard work—keep it short and sweet

253 Yes! Yesss! Yesssssssss!

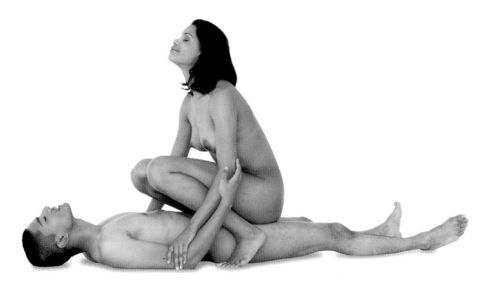

BEST FOR: when she wants to speed bounce on his shaft
HITS THE SPOT FOR: giving him an orgasmic massage
HOT TIP: it's a serious thigh workout. Start when you're both about to pop

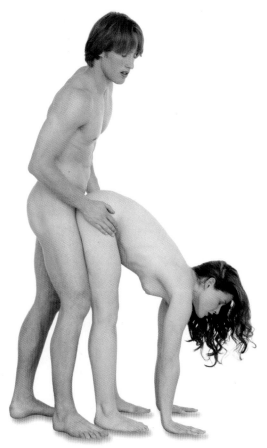

BEST FOR: when you wantonly surrender to sudden lust
HITS THE SPOT FOR: going in quick, fast, and deep
HOT TIP: guys—be firm and in control. She'll love it

255 Lounge lady

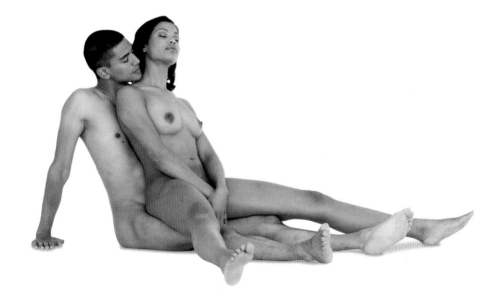

BEST FOR: couples who like playing manservant and lady
HITS THE SPOT FOR: the sexual turbo-charge of dominance and submission
HOT TIP: address her as "m'lady" at all times—and be obedient

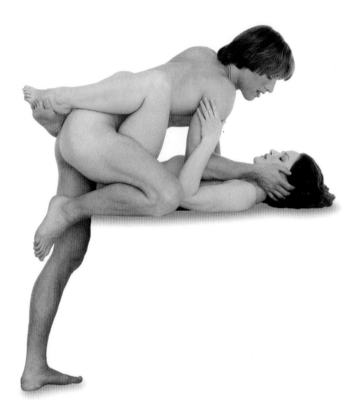

BEST FOR: sowing your seed
HITS THE SPOT FOR: plowing and furrowing
HOT TIP: don't worry about being dirty (but leave your boots at the door)

257 Passion fatigue

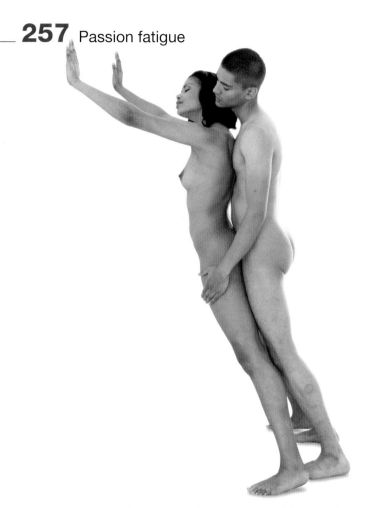

BEST FOR: when you've done it lots and you need that wall for support
HITS THE SPOT FOR: taking it slow and easy
HOT TIP: afterward, get into bed together and fall into a sex-satiated sleep

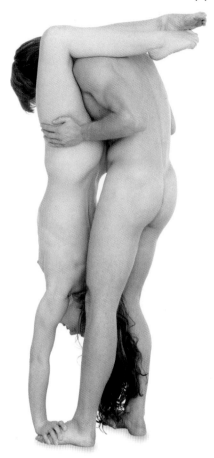

BEST FOR: women who can hold a handstand
HITS THE SPOT FOR: getting an exquisite faceful of her
HOT TIP: worried you won't look sexy upside down? Wear a corset

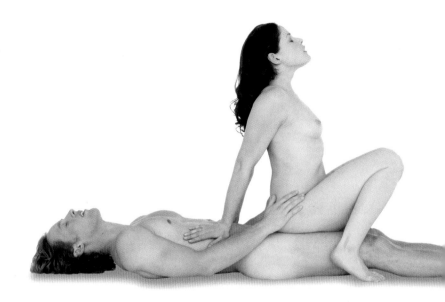

BEST FOR: third- or fourth-time-in-a-row sex
HITS THE SPOT FOR: forbidden and filthy fantasies
HOT TIP: throw your head back, push your chest out, and move

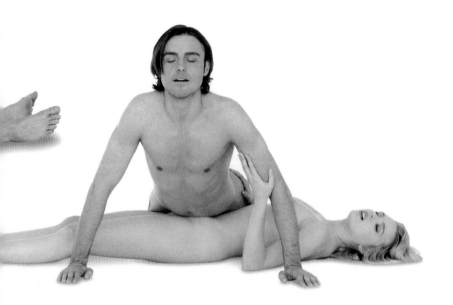

BEST FOR: some hot pre-sex thrusting between her thighs
HITS THE SPOT FOR: getting him hard, and her wet
HOT TIP: make yourselves slick with lube—now writhe like seals

261 The crush

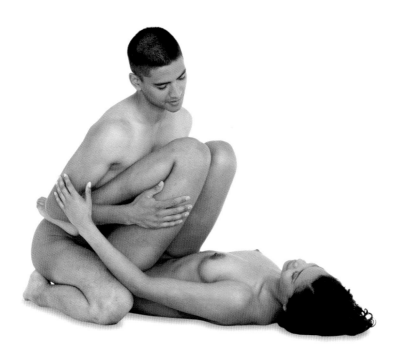

BEST FOR: when you want something long, slow, and sensual
HITS THE SPOT FOR: her feeling pleasurably crushed
HOT TIP: push her knees closer to her chest to max the sensation

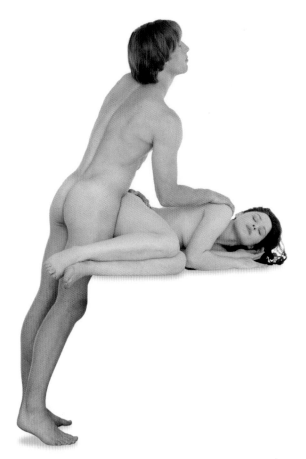

BEST FOR: when he works nights and she works days

HITS THE SPOT FOR: satisfying your lust in the overlap

HOT TIP: stroke her body and make all of your moves gentle

263 There's the rub

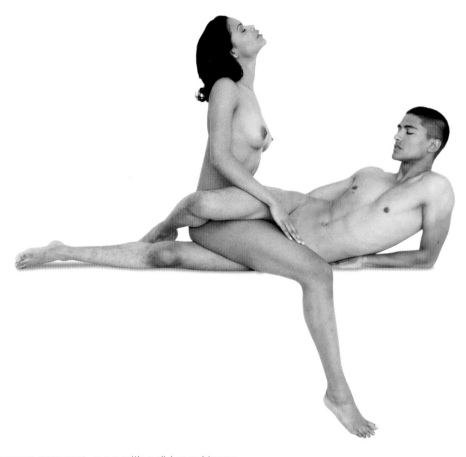

BEST FOR: guys with solid quadriceps
HITS THE SPOT FOR: tingles and tremors from sliding her clitoris on his thigh
HOT TIP: give her goose bumps by caressing her with a peacock feather

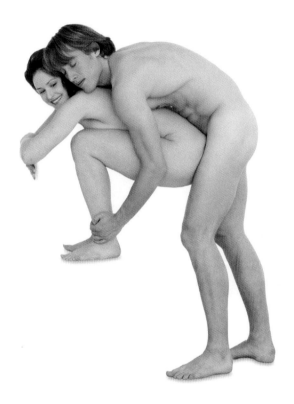

BEST FOR: powerful, macho sex with a big dose of intimacy
HITS THE SPOT FOR: her feeling wrapped up by him
HOT TIP: put your hands under her thighs and lift her up while you're inside

265 Snow white

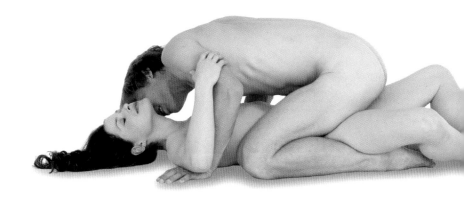

BEST FOR: love on a cold night
HITS THE SPOT FOR: steaming up the windows
HOT TIP: do it under a high-tog duvet

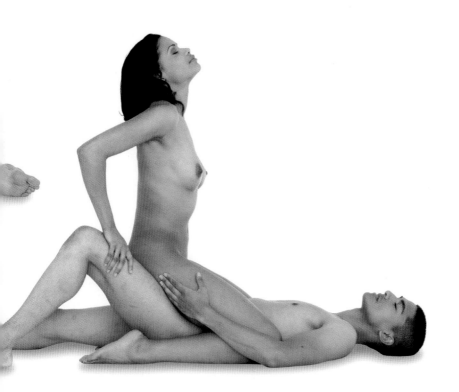

BEST FOR: celebrating her birthday
HITS THE SPOT FOR: free-form movement for her, plus a helping hand
HOT TIP: put down your champagne flutes before you start

267 Nice 'n' easy

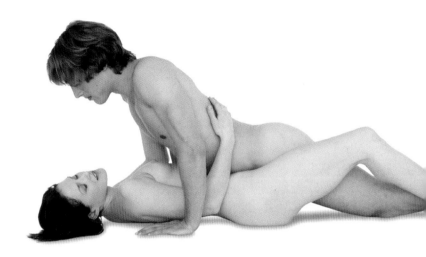

BEST FOR: good old-fashioned sex
HITS THE SPOT FOR: a thorough mattress pounding
HOT TIP: don't take your eyes off each other

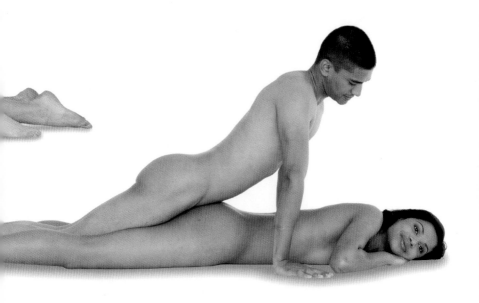

BEST FOR: bondage lovers ___
HITS THE SPOT FOR: delicious feelings of being restricted
HOT TIP: bind her wrists above her head

269 X & Y

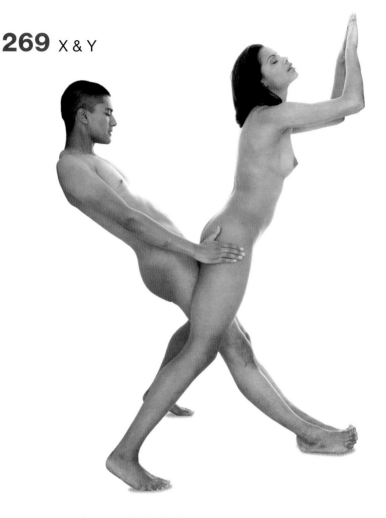

BEST FOR: goodbye sex in the hallway
HITS THE SPOT FOR: being the erotic alternative to a peck on the cheek
HOT TIP: kiss and walk away afterward. Don't speak

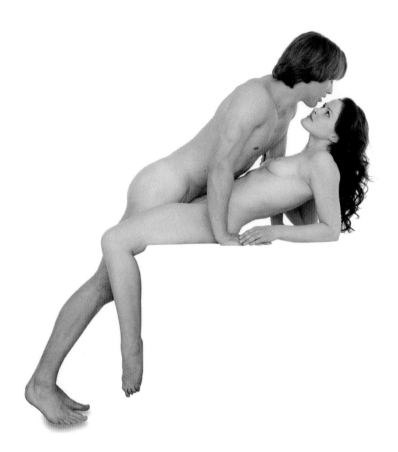

BEST FOR: Valentine's Day sex
HITS THE SPOT FOR: a heady cocktail of romance, lust, and go-for-it passion
HOT TIP: cover the bed in red rose petals (everyone should try it once)

271 Island of lust

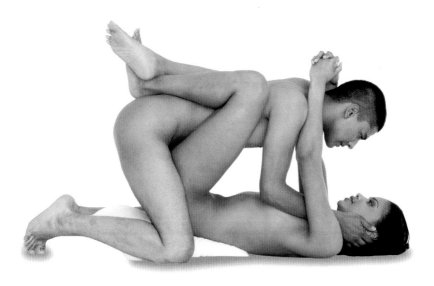

BEST FOR: those who like passionate leg locks
HITS THE SPOT FOR: sinking slowly into her
HOT TIP: carry her across the room and lay her on the bed in this position

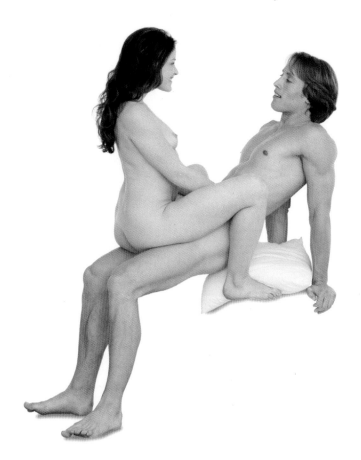

BEST FOR: when her sitting on his lap proves too much of a turn on
HITS THE SPOT FOR: frantic unzipping and skirt lifting, then "oh y-e-sss…"
HOT TIP: guys—take your weight on your hands and feet and get jiggy

273 Pythagoras in love

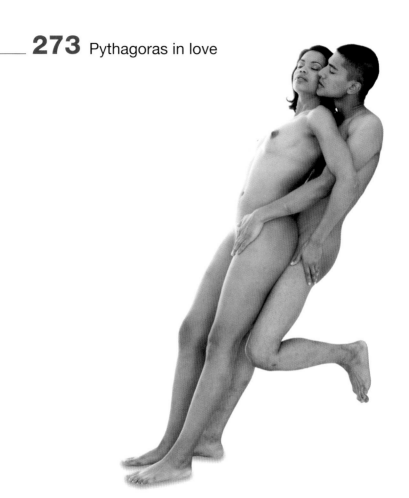

BEST FOR: couples with same-height genitals
HITS THE SPOT FOR: she feels warm, supported, and held from behind
HOT TIP: coat your palms in oil and slowly smooth them along her front

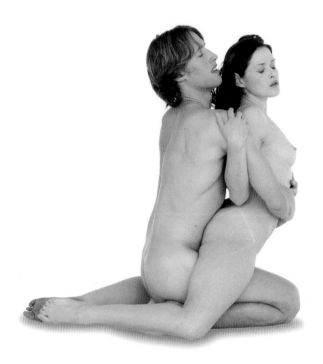

BEST FOR: when he wants to play the supporting role

HITS THE SPOT FOR: her feeling exquisitely stretched and taut

HOT TIP: pretend you're in *Titanic*

275 Perfect reunion

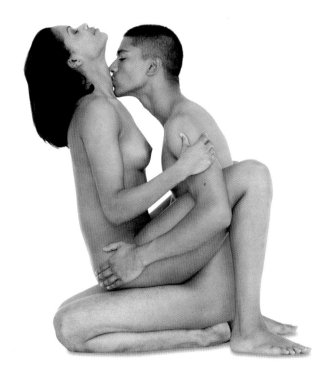

BEST FOR: when you want to kiss, nuzzle, and feed each other ice cream
HITS THE SPOT FOR: remembering why you're crazy about each other
HOT TIP: "accidentally" drop ice cream. Do the polite thing and lick it off

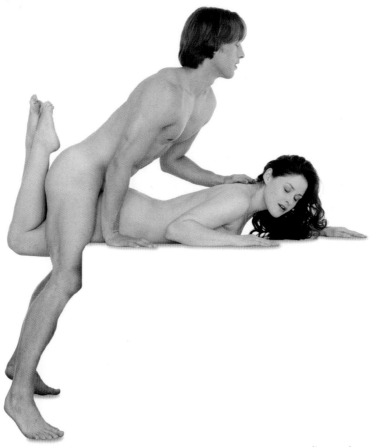

BEST FOR: sex opposite a mirror
HITS THE SPOT FOR: opening the door to anal sex
HOT TIP: go dressed for the occasion—a condom and a lot of lube

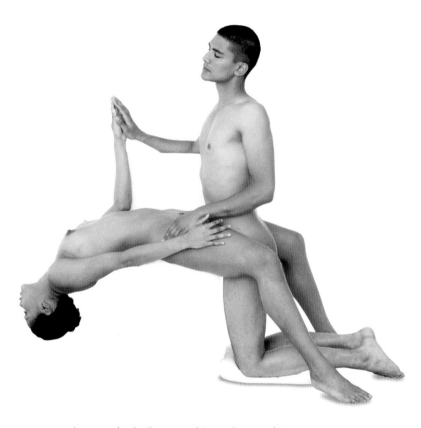

277 Melody maker

BEST FOR: when you're in the mood to make a noise
HITS THE SPOT FOR: stringing her body as tightly as a violin
HOT TIP: let rip with the sound—make it loud and guttural

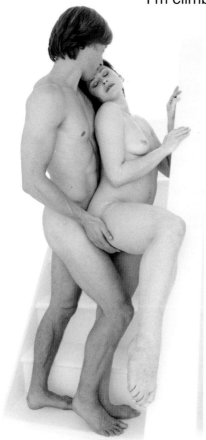

BEST FOR: when you need something solid to lean on
HITS THE SPOT FOR: sublime, knee-trembling naughtiness
HOT TIP: when you're finished, turn to look at each other and kiss

279 Honey, I'm home

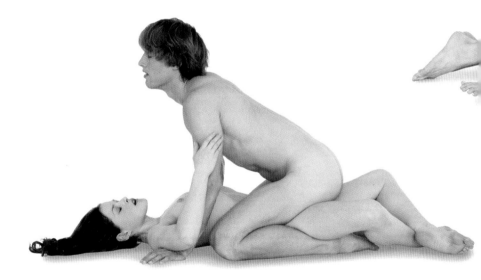

BEST FOR: the end of a l-o-n-g day
HITS THE SPOT FOR: making work seem like a distant memory
HOT TIP: it beats turning on the TV

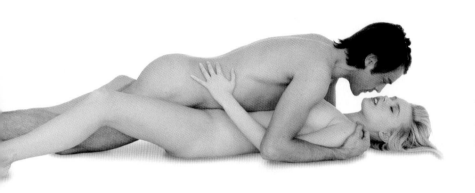

BEST FOR: sex when you're in the first throes of love
HITS THE SPOT FOR: a tight fit between your lips, tongues, and genitals
HOT TIP: passionate tongue-play essential

281 Old-timer

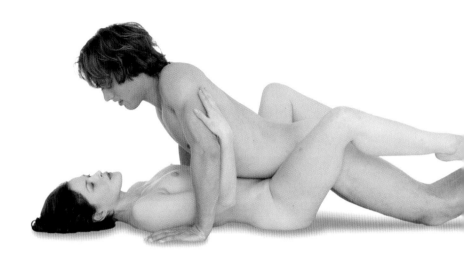
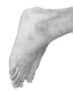

BEST FOR: no-nonsense sex when you haven't seen each other in a while
HITS THE SPOT FOR: getting straight down to business
HOT TIP: thrust to some sexy music

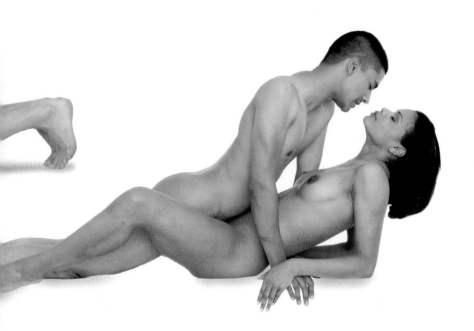

BEST FOR: second-time-in-a-row sex
HITS THE SPOT FOR: steamy, tummy-turning sensations
HOT TIP: try it on a chaise lounge

283 Tightly packaged

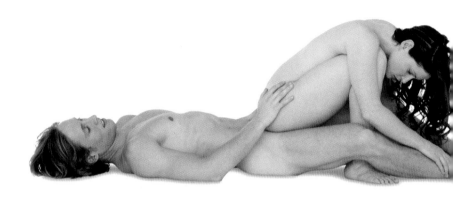

BEST FOR: carrying out ball-and-butt inspections
HITS THE SPOT FOR: guilt-free voyeurism
HOT TIP: caress his skin with your hair

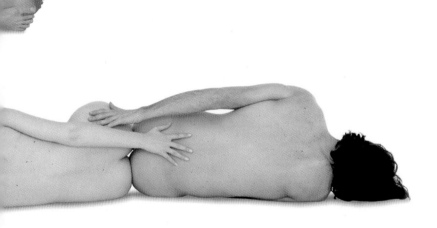

BEST FOR: when you're both tired
HITS THE SPOT FOR: staying connected with the option of later friskiness
HOT TIP: pop your hand through your thighs and stroke each other

285 Liquid ecstasy

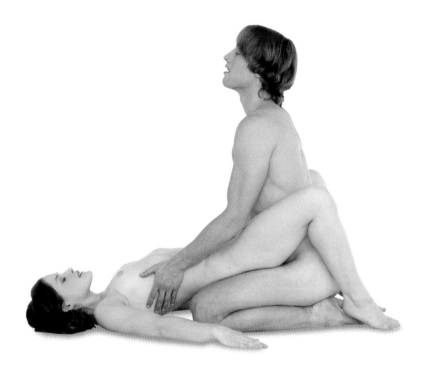

BEST FOR: sex meets erotic massage
HITS THE SPOT FOR: prolonging foreplay until you're bursting with desire
HOT TIP: when you're both ready, pull her onto you and go for it

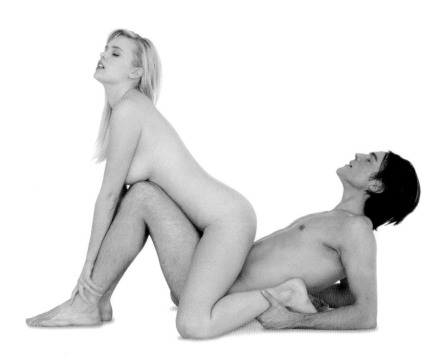

BEST FOR: when he wants to explore her anus with a well oiled finger
HITS THE SPOT FOR: adding the gasp factor to a saucy sex position
HOT TIP: women—the secret is to relax and enjoy down there

287 Passionate passenger

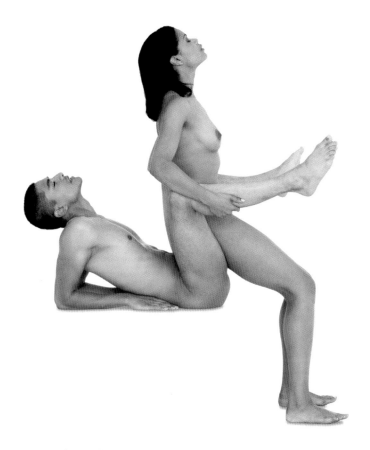

BEST FOR: the well-endowed man
HITS THE SPOT FOR: her sinking voluptuously onto his penis
HOT TIP: give him fast, slick, oral sex beforehand

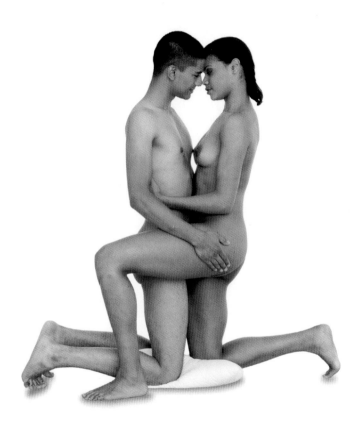

BEST FOR: tender, romantic moments
HITS THE SPOT FOR: gentle, barely-there caresses
HOT TIP: gently press your heads together and gaze into each other's eyes

289 Can you fit me in today?

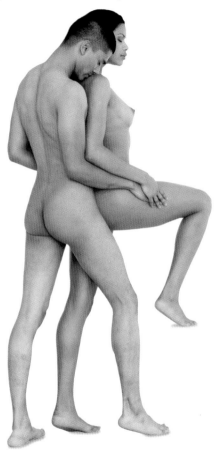

BEST FOR: when she's sliding off a stocking and he sidles up behind her
HITS THE SPOT FOR: making her feel like a sex kitten
HOT TIP: make it part of a strip show for him

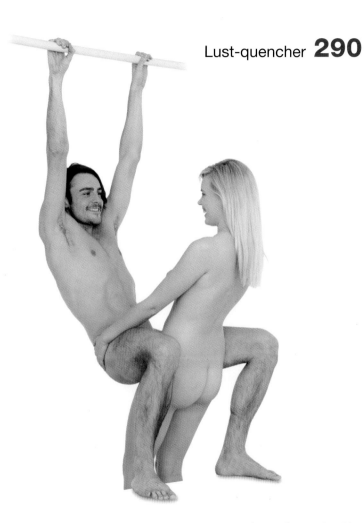

BEST FOR: sex where she carries him
HITS THE SPOT FOR: making you both feel brazenly horny
HOT TIP: grab his ass and move him at the speed you like

291 Strangers in the night

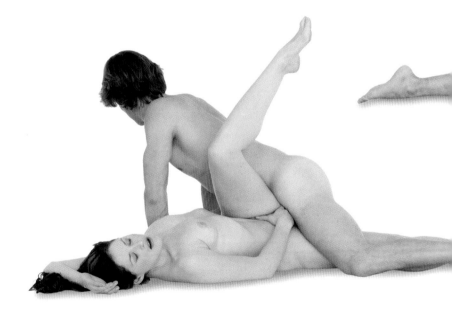

BEST FOR: when intimacy's not important
HITS THE SPOT FOR: getting swept away by sexy thoughts
HOT TIP: make his buttock tingle with an unexpected spank

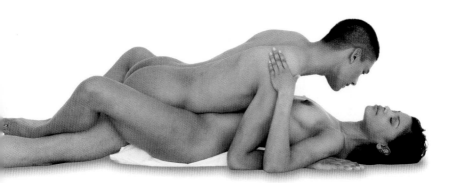

BEST FOR: when you don't want anything fancy
HITS THE SPOT FOR: him taking charge of things
HOT TIP: a pillow or cushion underneath her will "raise the seat of pleasure"

293 Take a bow

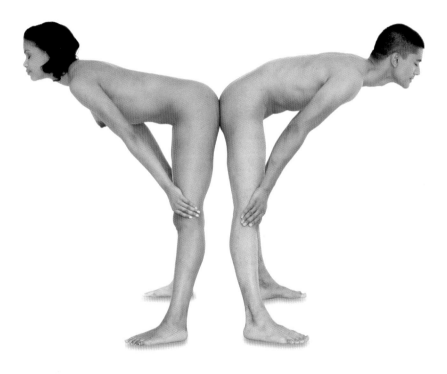

BEST FOR: improbable sex (or, if you're kinky, using a double-ended dildo)
HITS THE SPOT FOR: buttock rubbing
HOT TIP: stand up, turn around, and take her from behind

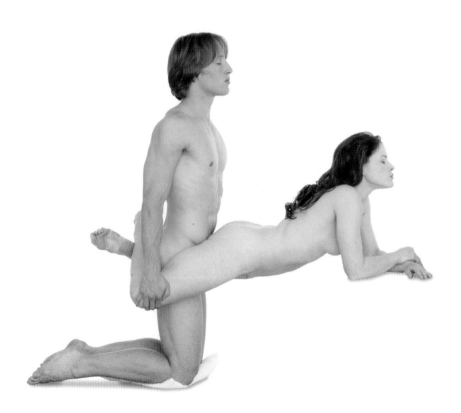

BEST FOR: when he wants to meet her every need
HITS THE SPOT FOR: making her garden feel tended
HOT TIP: act servile — she's the lady of the house

295 The quest

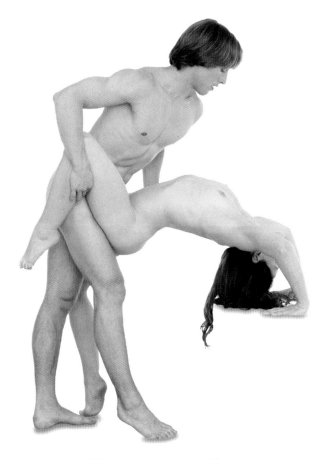

BEST FOR: lovers who will bend over backward for pleasure
HITS THE SPOT FOR: electric sensations that zip up and down your bodies
HOT TIP: afterward lean over, pick her up, and carry her to bed

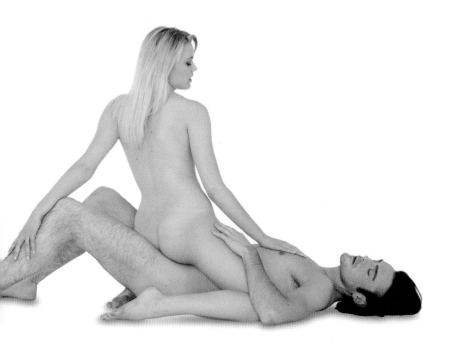

BEST FOR: her-on-top sex, but with a side twist
HITS THE SPOT FOR: a rousing angle between his pubic bone and her clitoris
HOT TIP: move like you're being bounced on a gently trotting pony

297 Private tutor

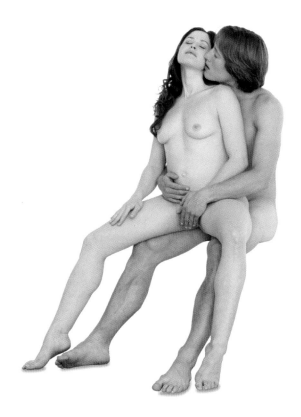

BEST FOR: her-to-him masturbation tutorials
HITS THE SPOT FOR: teaching him strokes that make her hair stand on end
HOT TIP: masturbate while he watches—purely for educational purposes

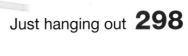

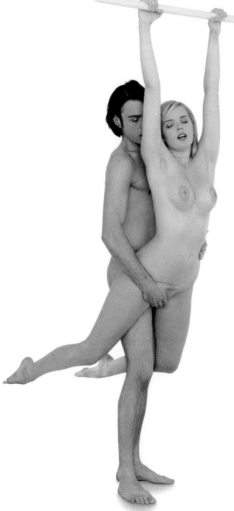

BEST FOR: after a visit to Cirque du Soleil
HITS THE SPOT FOR: delicious his-hand-on-her-clitoris sensations
HOT TIP: strong pole needed (in more ways than one)

299 The handmaiden

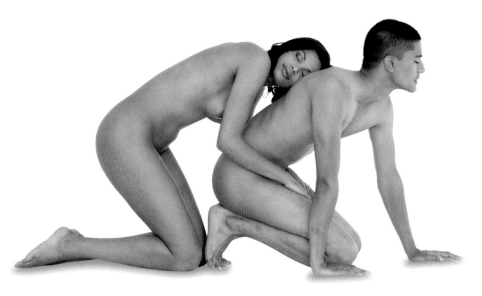

BEST FOR: letting him know you want him
HITS THE SPOT FOR: gentle hand caresses from behind
HOT TIP: press your breasts and lips against his back

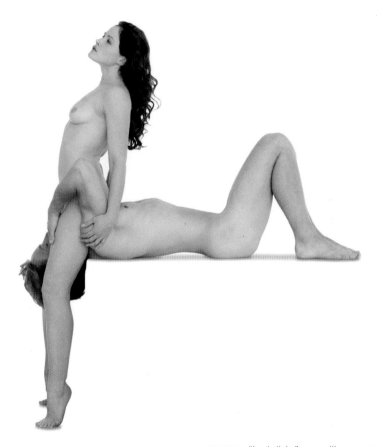

BEST FOR: "invisible" cunnilingus

HITS THE SPOT FOR: tongue teasing until she can't stand it any more

HOT TIP: squeeze her clitoris with your index and middle fingers—now lick

301 The job interview

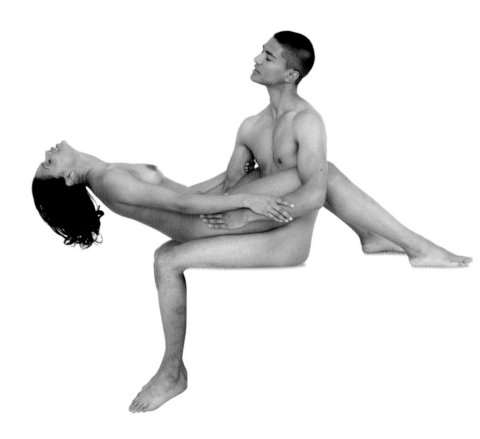

BEST FOR: when you want to assess each other's sex skills
HITS THE SPOT FOR: making you extra eager to impress
HOT TIP: ask: "what do you think you can bring to this position?"

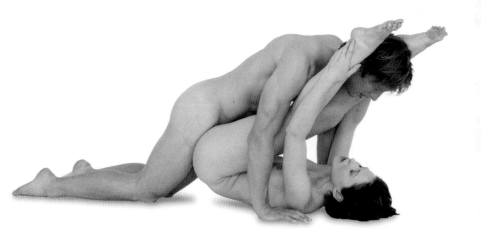

BEST FOR: the morning after the night before
HITS THE SPOT FOR: getting the blood rushing around your bodies
HOT TIP: go out for brunch afterward

303 Kneeling at the altar

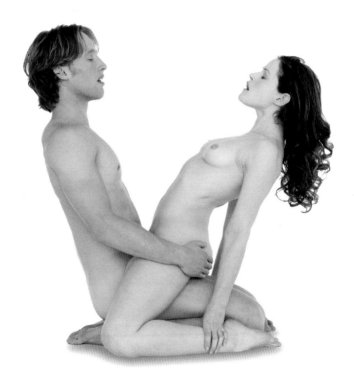

BEST FOR: easy, deep, face-to-face sex
HITS THE SPOT FOR: worshiping each other's body
HOT TIP: use your lips, teeth, and tongue on each other

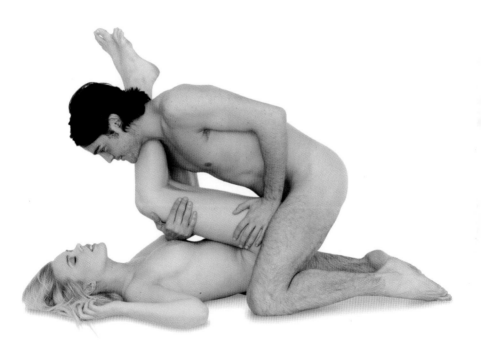

BEST FOR: when you're overtaken by irrepressible lust

HITS THE SPOT FOR: waking up the neighbors

HOT TIP: move like you mean it

305 I'm not done with you

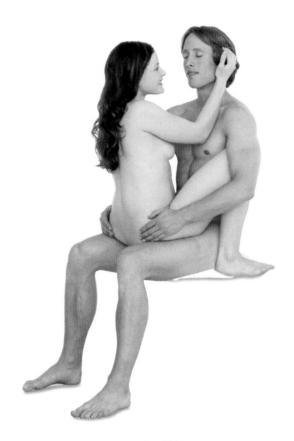

BEST FOR: when she can't get enough of him
HITS THE SPOT FOR: making him feel like sex on legs
HOT TIP: keep going until you pass out

Do you come here often? **306**

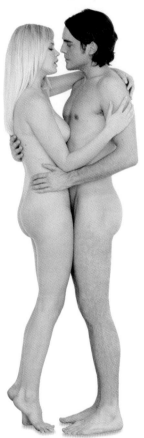

BEST FOR: thrusting between her thighs

HITS THE SPOT FOR: plenty of back-and-forth friction on her clitoris

HOT TIP: chat away like nothing's happening down below

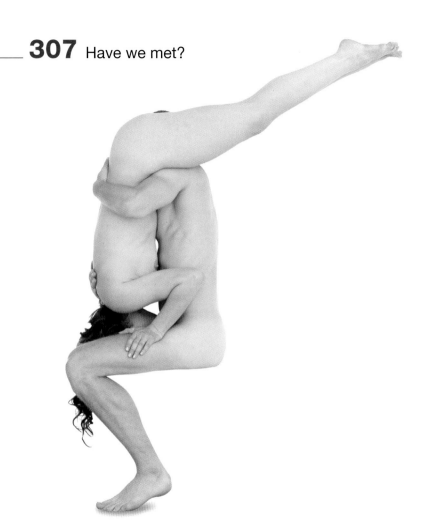

307 Have we met?

BEST FOR: when she's head over heels
HITS THE SPOT FOR: a cuddle meets upside-down lip service
HOT TIP: if it's all a bit hit and miss, lie back and do it the conventional way

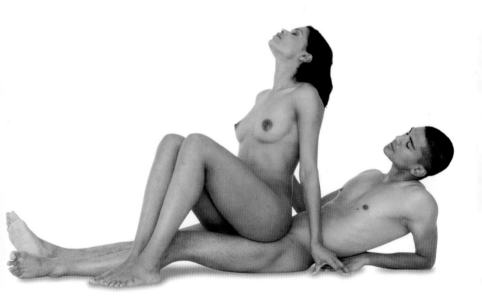

BEST FOR: a heavenly start to the day

HITS THE SPOT FOR: making the most of his early morning hard-on

HOT TIP: share breakfast in bed afterward

309 Lowering the tone

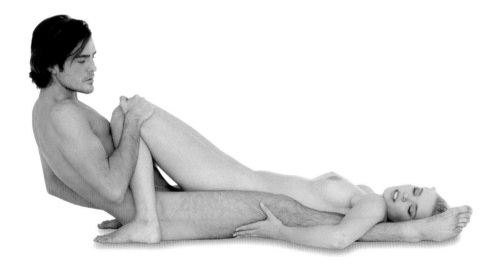

BEST FOR: when you want an excuse to avoid the gym
HITS THE SPOT FOR: toning your abs on the job
HOT TIP: men—lower yourself all the way to the ground and up again

Running for President **310**

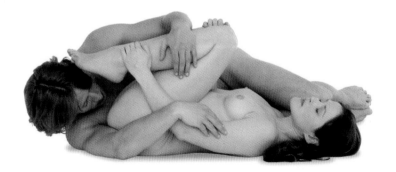

BEST FOR: when he's aiming to please
HITS THE SPOT FOR: being a sure-fire winner among women voters
HOT TIP: now's no time for delicate licks—get your face wet

311 Ankle brace

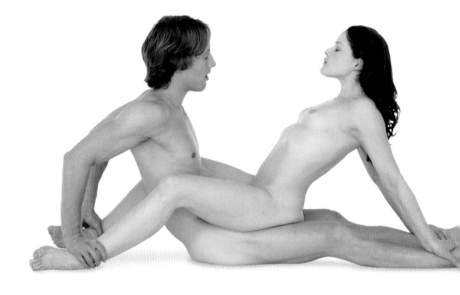

BEST FOR: when you want to get a grip on each other
HITS THE SPOT FOR: trapping each other in position
HOT TIP: say: "I won't let go unless you do"

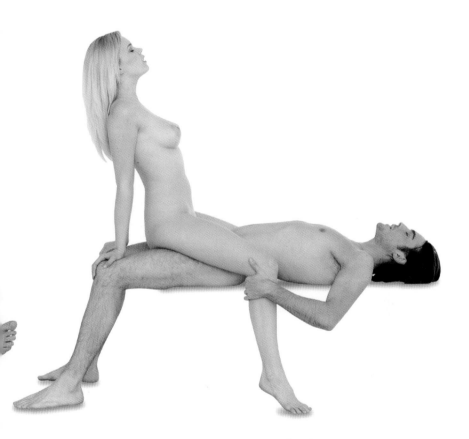

BEST FOR: pleasing both sides equally
HITS THE SPOT FOR: the freedom of clitoris access for her
HOT TIP: girls – stand up slightly and make circles with your bottom

313 Ballet practice

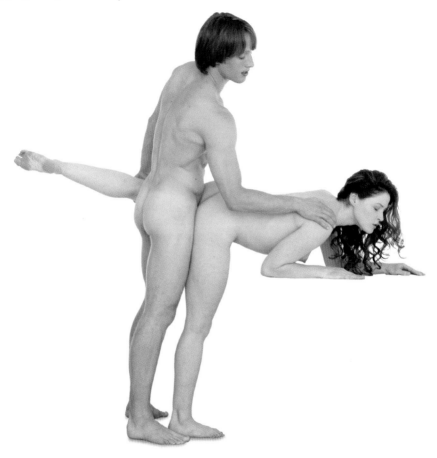

BEST FOR: strong and streamlined penetration
HITS THE SPOT FOR: knowing you look graceful when you're on the job
HOT TIP: girls—best not to do this in heels

Drag him out unconscious 314

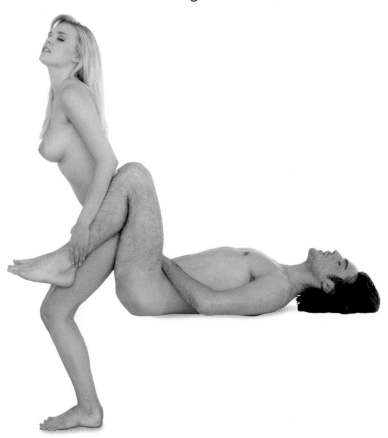

BEST FOR: when he's barely capable
HITS THE SPOT FOR: the power trip of her bobbing up and down on him
HOT TIP: it's easier if his feet are on the floor

315 Lust generator

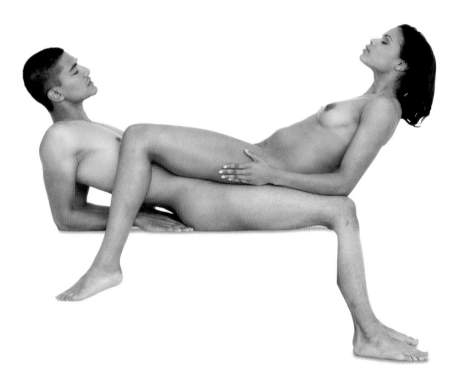

BEST FOR: when you're in the mood for a laid-back beginning
HITS THE SPOT FOR: building up lust until you're both on fire
HOT TIP: girls – meet his eye, then slowly bend forward and kiss him

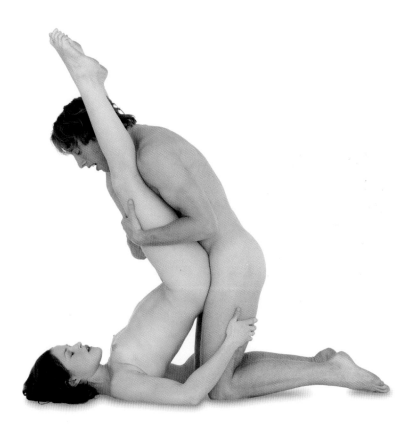

BEST FOR: the caffeine-free way of kick-starting the morning

HITS THE SPOT FOR: feeling invigorated afterwards

HOT TIP: don't try it on a waterbed

317 Take a seat madam

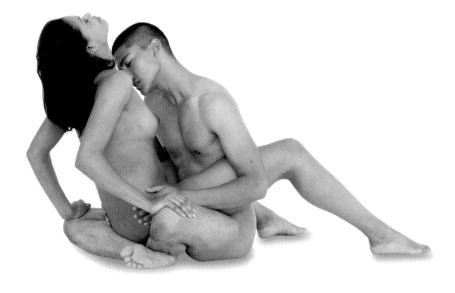

BEST FOR: warm, friendly, companionable sex
HITS THE SPOT FOR: kissing and neck nuzzling
HOT TIP: hold each other's head in your hands

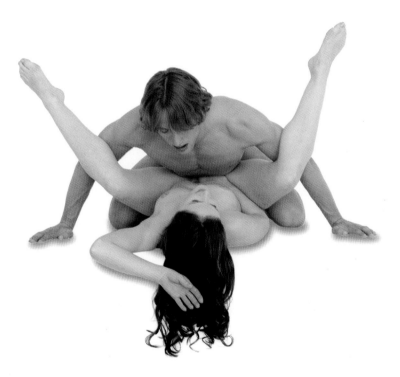

BEST FOR: wannabe porn stars
HITS THE SPOT FOR: the thrill of performing
HOT TIP: go the true exhibitionist route and film yourselves

319 Whirlwind romance

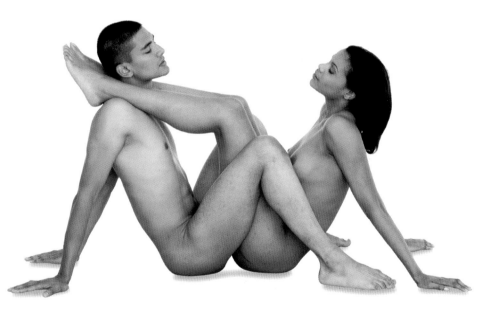

BEST FOR: sex when there's no time to lose
HITS THE SPOT FOR: frenzied pushing and banging to make your head spin
HOT TIP: do it till the crack of dawn

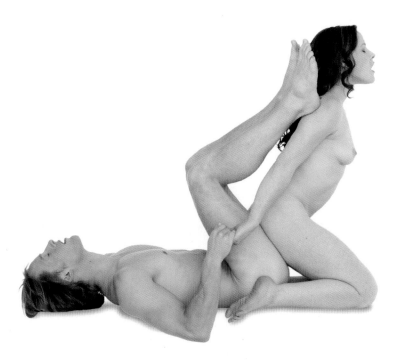

BEST FOR: when he wants to lie back and put his feet up
HITS THE SPOT FOR: letting your fantasies take over
HOT TIP: girls—grind your bottom against him

321 The tip-off

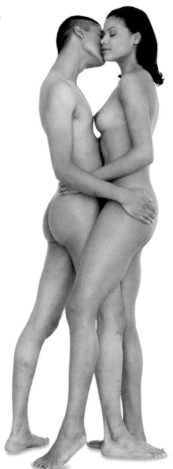

BEST FOR: whetting the erotic appetite
HITS THE SPOT FOR: very shallow penetration by the tip of his penis
HOT TIP: girls — try wearing heels

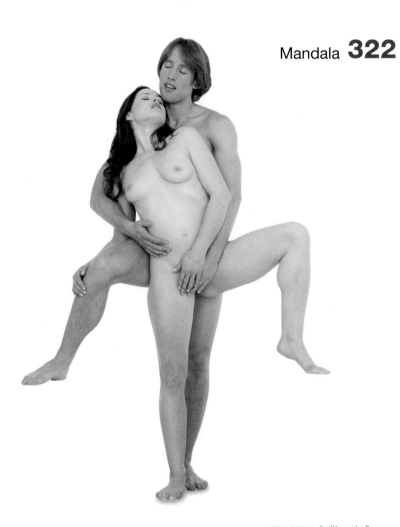

Mandala **322**

BEST FOR: "cliterate" men
HITS THE SPOT FOR: a customized, by-hand orgasm
HOT TIP: a guiding hand on top of his will tell him all he needs to know

323 On tonight's menu

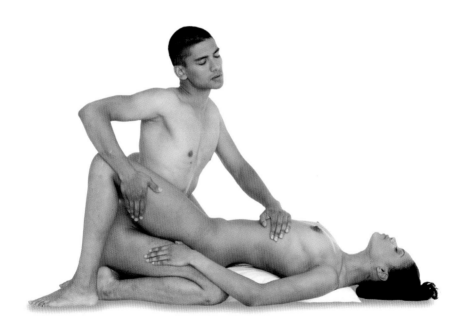

BEST FOR: when you're feeling hungry for love and hungry for food
HITS THE SPOT FOR: drizzling her body with honey (or anything lickable)
HOT TIP: use her navel as a honey pot—delve into it with your tongue

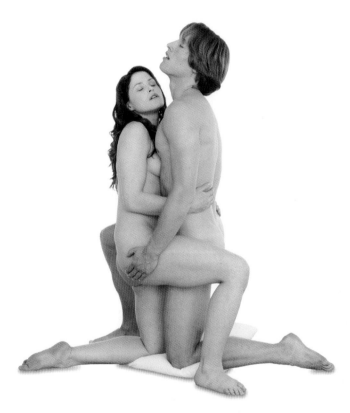

BEST FOR: celebrating your engagement
HITS THE SPOT FOR: losing yourself in a passionate kiss
HOT TIP: whisper sweet nothings to each other

325 Please enter quietly

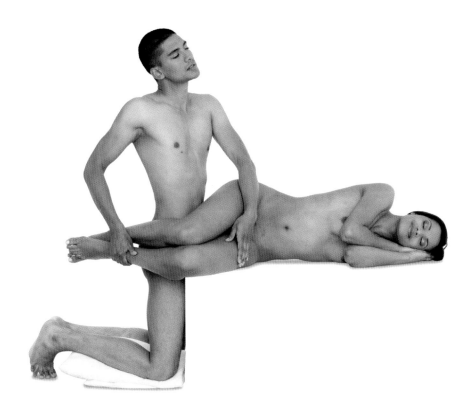

BEST FOR: when he wants to have sex but she's sleepy
HITS THE SPOT FOR: being intimate while he does all the work
HOT TIP: cuddle in the spoons position afterward

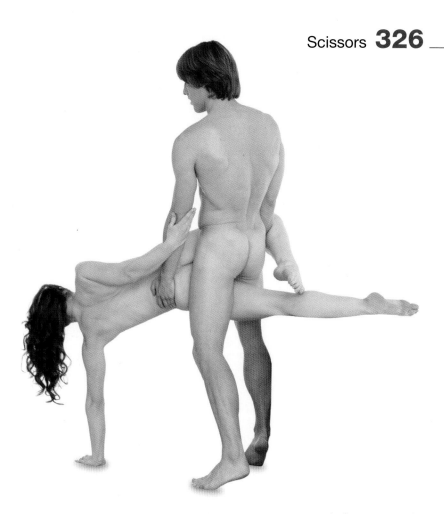

BEST FOR: trainee gymnasts
HITS THE SPOT FOR: a unique, acrobatic angle of penetration
HOT TIP: if it all gets too much, take a breather in the doggie position

327 Stargazing

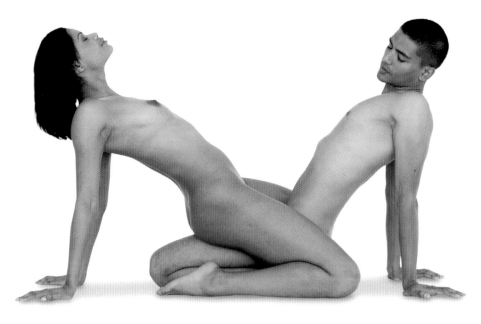

BEST FOR: taking a quick breather
HITS THE SPOT FOR: shared quiet moments
HOT TIP: who says mirrored ceilings are cheesy?

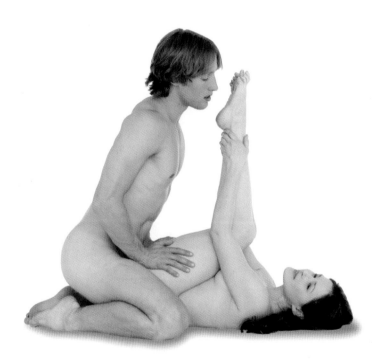

BEST FOR: men who have a thing for feet
HITS THE SPOT FOR: losing yourself in sensation
HOT TIP: whisper your lover's name (who cares if it's corny?)

329 Laptop

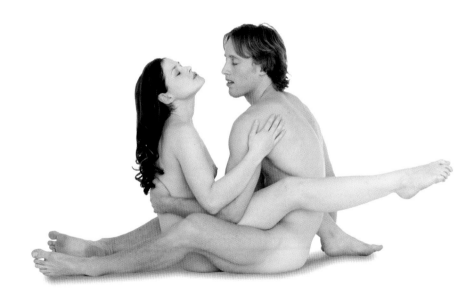

BEST FOR: after-dinner sex
HITS THE SPOT FOR: upright movements without too much belly bumping
HOT TIP: pass an after-dinner mint back and forth between your mouths

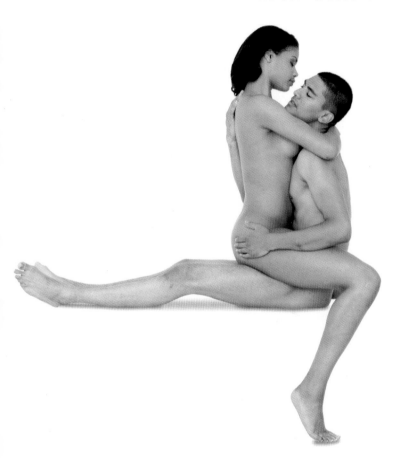

BEST FOR: get-well-soon sex
HITS THE SPOT FOR: her giving him his medicine
HOT TIP: girls — wear a nurse's uniform; guys — go naked

331 Pyramid of passion

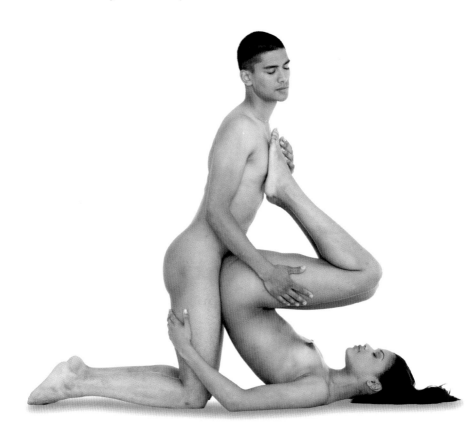

BEST FOR: when you want feverish intensity
HITS THE SPOT FOR: bed shaking and earth moving
HOT TIP: strong sensations guaranteed—make sure you're warmed up first

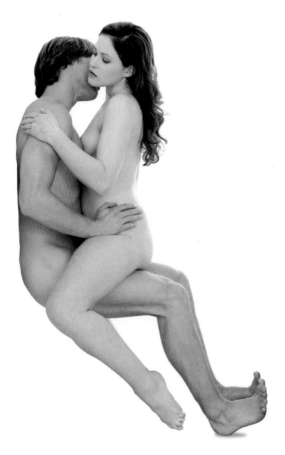

BEST FOR: unexpected alleyway and toilet stall sex ——————
HITS THE SPOT FOR: delighting in sudden speedy sex
HOT TIP: press against each other and make out like teenagers

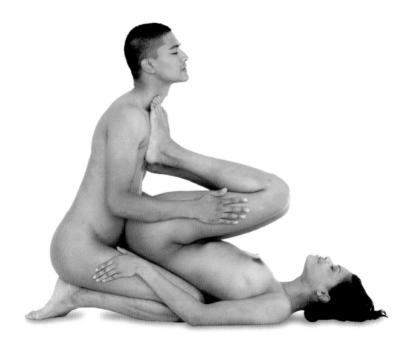

BEST FOR: high-octane, high-impact sex
HITS THE SPOT FOR: vibrations that rock your body
HOT TIP: she can vary the sensations by hooking her legs over his shoulders

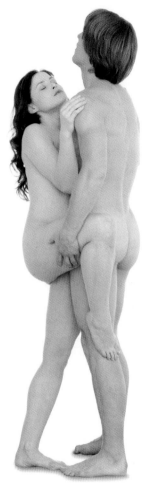

BEST FOR: spur-of-the-moment sex _____
HITS THE SPOT FOR: letting raw passion overwhelm you
HOT TIP: guys—part your legs for a stable base

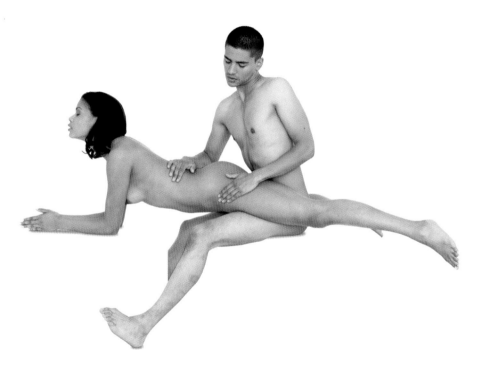

BEST FOR: nooky in front of the TV
HITS THE SPOT FOR: turbo-charged arousal while watching an X-rated movie
HOT TIP: have your adult toybox at hand

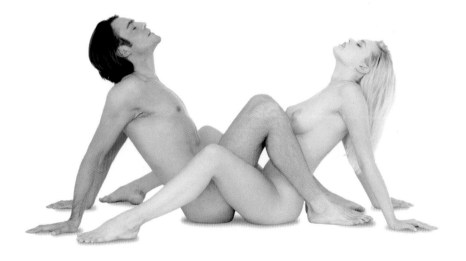

BEST FOR: when you want a mid-sex chat
HITS THE SPOT FOR: friendliness rather than sizzling passion
HOT TIP: don't expect deep penetration

337 Holy poker

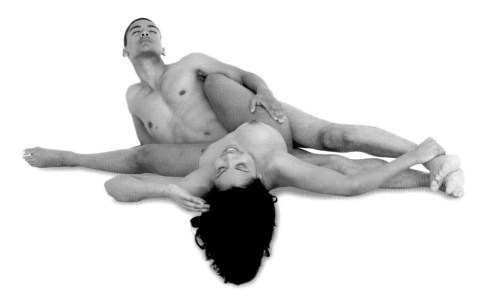

BEST FOR: sex that looks casual but feels intense
HITS THE SPOT FOR: making you shudder with desire
HOT TIP: guys—try moving in slow motion

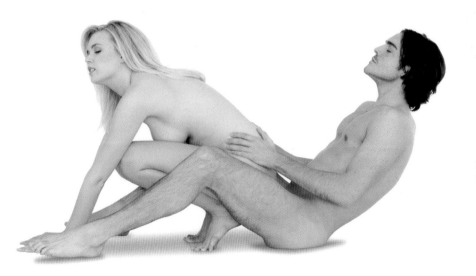

BEST FOR: hot, wet, and bubbly bath sex
HITS THE SPOT FOR: getting dirty and clean at the same time
HOT TIP: bubble bath and candles essential

339 The big night

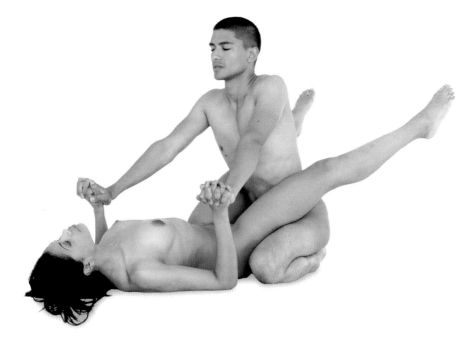

BEST FOR: Saturday night sex
HITS THE SPOT FOR: enjoying those let's-just-hump moments
HOT TIP: girls—wear red hooker-style heels

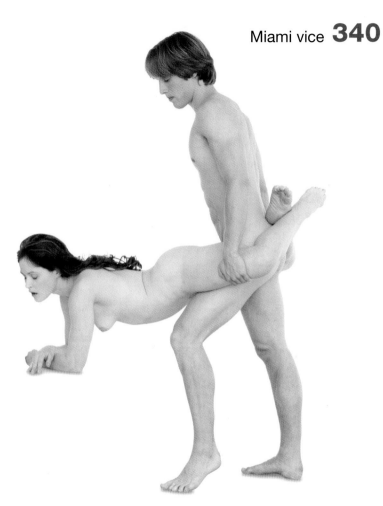

BEST FOR: girls who are good at balancing, gripping, and squeezing
HITS THE SPOT FOR: checking another tricky sexploit off the list
HOT TIP: give him a firm "handshake" (a vice-like grip with your vagina)

341 Hot-desking

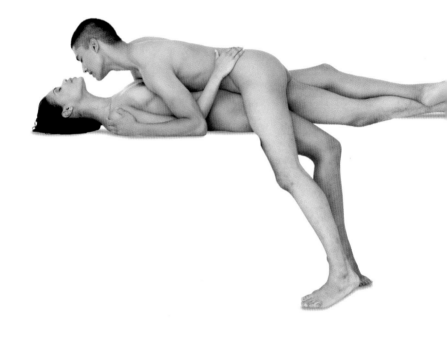

BEST FOR: sex in the office (check that no one else is "working late")
HITS THE SPOT FOR: making a tough day at work seem all worthwhile
HOT TIP: check out the security camera footage afterward

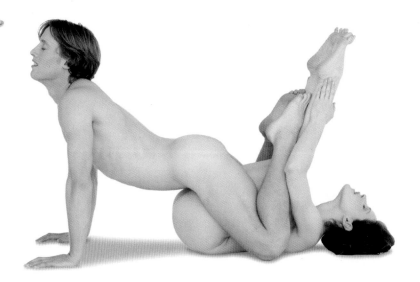

BEST FOR: lovers in search of innovation
HITS THE SPOT FOR: being close yet distant
HOT TIP: write about it in your sex blog

343 Princess on the throne

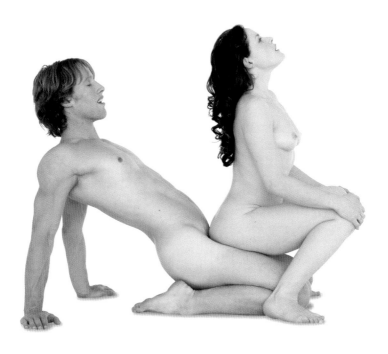

BEST FOR: when she needs a sit-down
HITS THE SPOT FOR: intense "G-on-G" (glans on G-spot) sensations
HOT TIP: make her shiver by flexing the muscles at the base of your penis

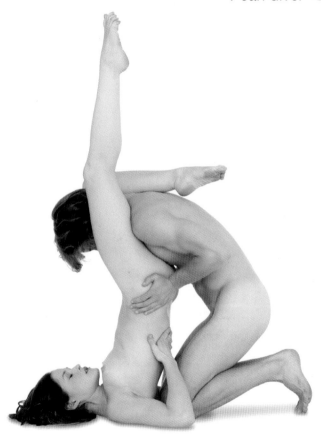

BEST FOR: when she likes to watch
HITS THE SPOT FOR: blissfully winding your tongue around her clitoris
HOT TIP: guys—make it clear that this is your favorite thing in the world

345 Yacht on a calm sea

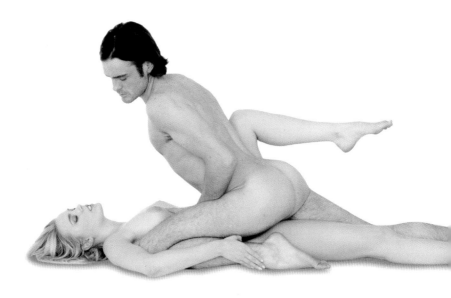

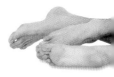

BEST FOR: seriously sleek sex
HITS THE SPOT FOR: gliding smoothly in and out
HOT TIP: run the tip of your tongue provocatively around your lips

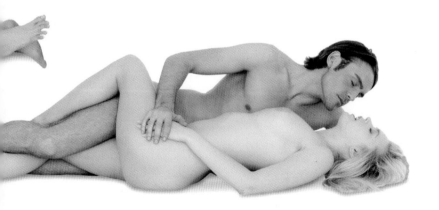

BEST FOR: sex inside a sleeping bag
HITS THE SPOT FOR: feeling warm, close, and intertwined
HOT TIP: festival-goers—don't rely on the band to disguise your moans

347 Bar job

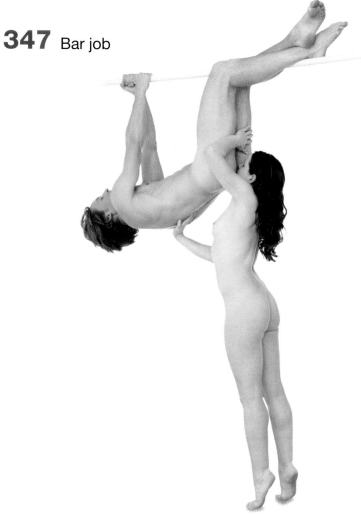

BEST FOR: high-octane bottom love
HITS THE SPOT FOR: tongue action that will make him gasp
HOT TIP: give him a cheeky love bite while you're there

The hotseat **348**

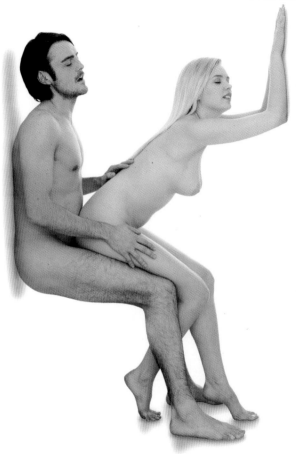

BEST FOR: when you want strong thighs for your next ski trip
HITS THE SPOT FOR: intense sensation that will bring tears to her eyes
HOT TIP: if your thighs can't take it, have a stool on standby

349 Upside down you're turning me

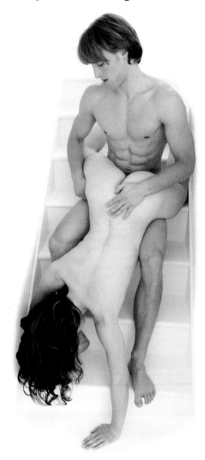

BEST FOR: thrills-on-the-stairs seekers
HITS THE SPOT FOR: turning a sedate sex life on its head
HOT TIP: penetration might be difficult, but finger power won't be

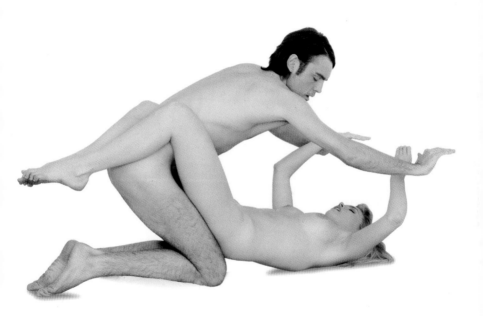

BEST FOR: moments of burning desire
HITS THE SPOT FOR: taking you gasping to the finish line
HOT TIP: brace yourself against the headboard and go for it

351 Leg lock

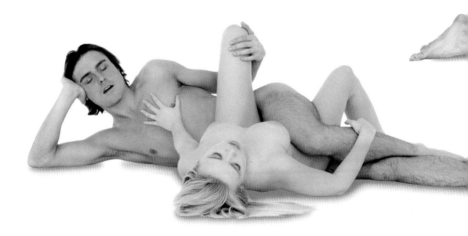

BEST FOR: a new line in side-on sex
HITS THE SPOT FOR: feeling trapped (in a good way)
HOT TIP: boys—cock that upper leg when you wanna move

Pull hitter **352**

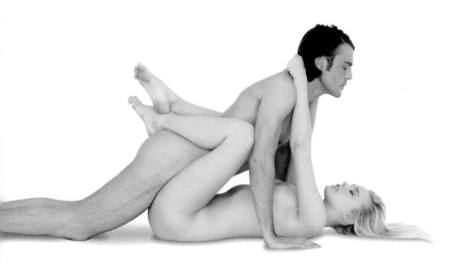

BEST FOR: when she wants to grab him and pull him into her
HITS THE SPOT FOR: showing the force of her desire
HOT TIP: cross your ankles and pull your body up to meet his

353 Sausage sandwich

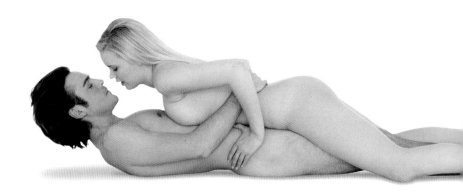
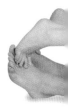

BEST FOR: when you've just had sex and you want a repeat performance
HITS THE SPOT FOR: feeling him get hard a second time
HOT TIP: let the tension build to snapping point before you start to move

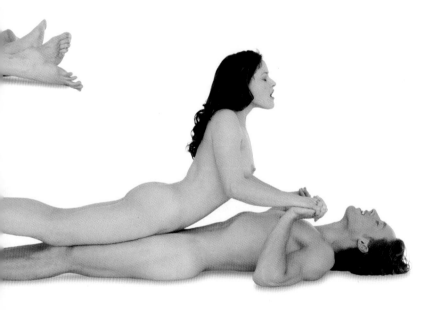

BEST FOR: women who find the big O elusive during sex
HITS THE SPOT FOR: pushing and grinding her clitoris against his hard parts
HOT TIP: forget thrusting (for now) and concentrate on friction

355 Wuthering heights

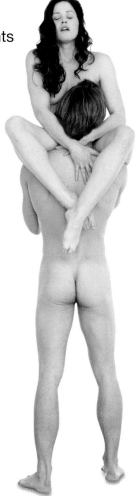

BEST FOR: couples who get high on cunnilingus
HITS THE SPOT FOR: erotic head shakes on her bits (as if he's saying "no!")
HOT TIP: caution! Surround yourself by soft surfaces

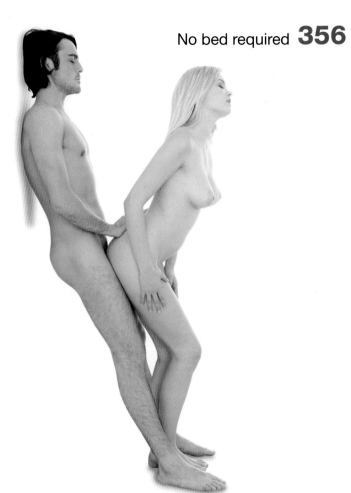

BEST FOR: "excuse us, we have some business in the next room" sex
HITS THE SPOT FOR: escaping from something boring to something exciting
HOT TIP: give each other speed-oral sex beforehand

357 The raft

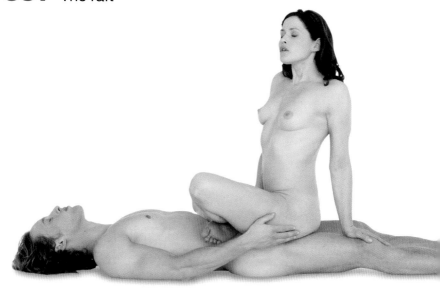

BEST FOR: when you want to practice your tantric breathing
HITS THE SPOT FOR: opening your chakras
HOT TIP: play a recording of waves lapping on a shore

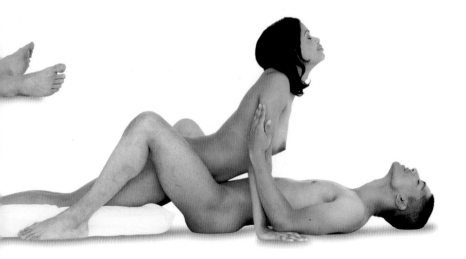

BEST FOR: when she wants to rub his stiff bits

HITS THE SPOT FOR: giving and getting a full frontal massage

HOT TIP: breasts are great massage tools

359 Sweet as sugar

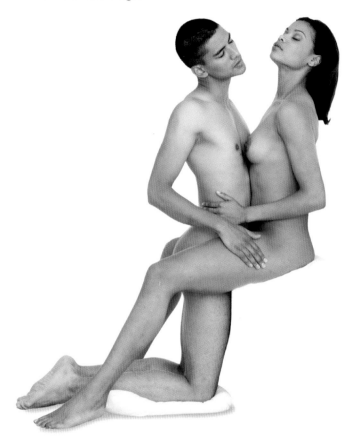

BEST FOR: touchy-feely love
HITS THE SPOT FOR: soft kisses and gentle caresses
HOT TIP: play your favorite love song

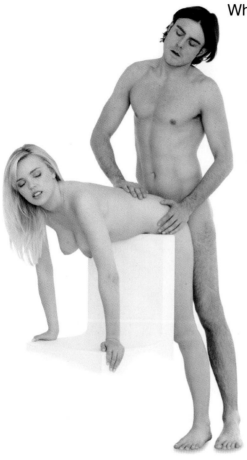

Wham! Bam! 360

BEST FOR: rip-each-other's-clothes-off sex
HITS THE SPOT FOR: expressing the unrestrained animal in you
HOT TIP: be tender and lovey dovey afterward

361 Tight squeeze

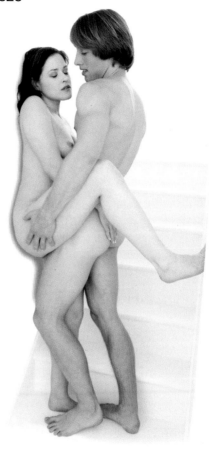

BEST FOR: seedy sex in corridors and stairwells
HITS THE SPOT FOR: some solid thrusting without the risk of falling over
HOT TIP: women, tilt your pelvis forward; it'll make things a whole lot easier

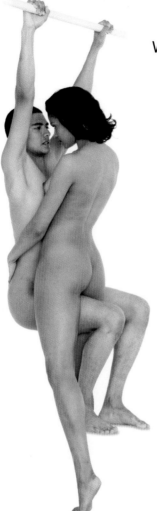

BEST FOR: acrobat wannabes
HITS THE SPOT FOR: some climax-clinching frottage
HOT TIP: slowly press your thigh deeply into her

363 I only came to fix the TV

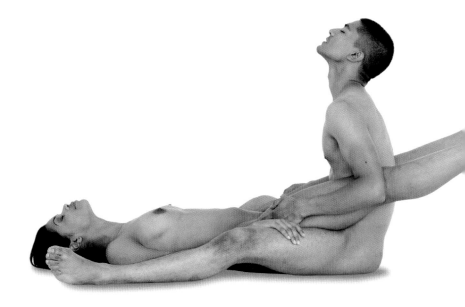

BEST FOR: the "repairman seduced by housewife" role play
HITS THE SPOT FOR: fiddling with her buttons instead
HOT TIP: guys—remember to bring a wide range of tools

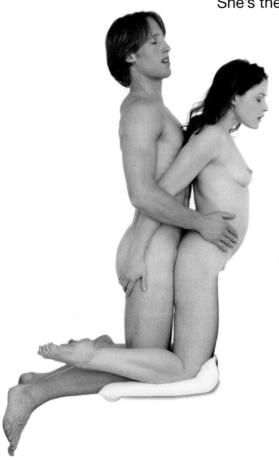

BEST FOR: sex in the back row of the movie theater
HITS THE SPOT FOR: the thrill of sex in the same room as Cameron Diaz
HOT TIP: make sure it's a private screening

365 Girl overboard

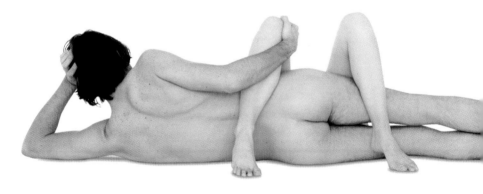

BEST FOR: when she's just collapsed on the bed with lust
HITS THE SPOT FOR: a "When Harry Met Sally" style orgasm
HOT TIP: guys—if she's making the right sounds, DON'T STOP

now it's time to start
all over again…

When you're in the mood for...Fast and furious

Heady, passion-fueled ways to pump and grind.

When you're in the mood for...Slow and sensual

Positions to gradually build up the pressure to a mind-blowing climax.

When you're in the mood for…Acrobatics

For superior sexperts, positions to help you show off your skills.

When you're in the mood for...Sexercise

Orgasmic ways to work those thighs and tone those abs—you'll never need to go to the gym again.

When you're in the mood for...Romance

For those tender moments, when you want to feel warm and fuzzy with your lover.

When you're in the mood for...Impromtu encounters

Easy access for when lust strikes, wherever you are...

When you're in the mood for...Funny and frisky

Fodder for some real sexperimentation, but don't take yourselves too seriously, and giggle if it goes wrong.

When you're in the mood for...Nice n'easy

Classic tried-and-tested positions that don't require backs of steel or elastic limbs.

Acknowledgements
DK would like to thank Lynne Brown, Fergus Muir,
and Susie Adams for arranging photography.